NOLS Backcountry Nutrition

Eating Beyond the Basics

Mary Howley Ryan, MS, RD

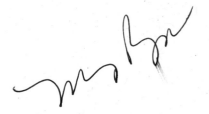

STACKPOLE
BOOKS

Published by
STACKPOLE BOOKS
5067 Ritter Road
Mechanicsburg, PA 17055
www.stackpolebooks.com

Printed in the United States

First edition

10 9 8 7 6 5 4 3 2 1

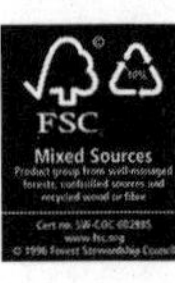

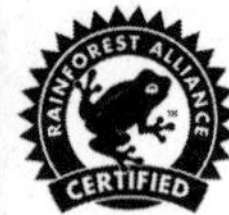

This book was printed using responsible environmental practices by FSC-certified book manufacturers. The Forest Stewardship Council encourages the responsible management of the world's forests. The Rainforest Alliance works to conserve biodiversity and ensure sustainable livelihoods by transforming land-use practices, business practices, and consumer behavior.

Library of Congress Cataloging-in-Publication Data

Ryan, Mary Howley.
NOLS backcountry nutrition : eating beyond the basics / Mary Howley Ryan.
p. cm.
Includes bibliographical references and index.
ISBN-13: 978-0-8117-3505-6 (alk. paper)
ISBN-10: 0-8117-3505-2 (alk. paper)
1. Outdoor life. 2. Nutrition. I. Title.
TX823.R933 2008
613.2—dc22

2008003806

Contents

List of Tables

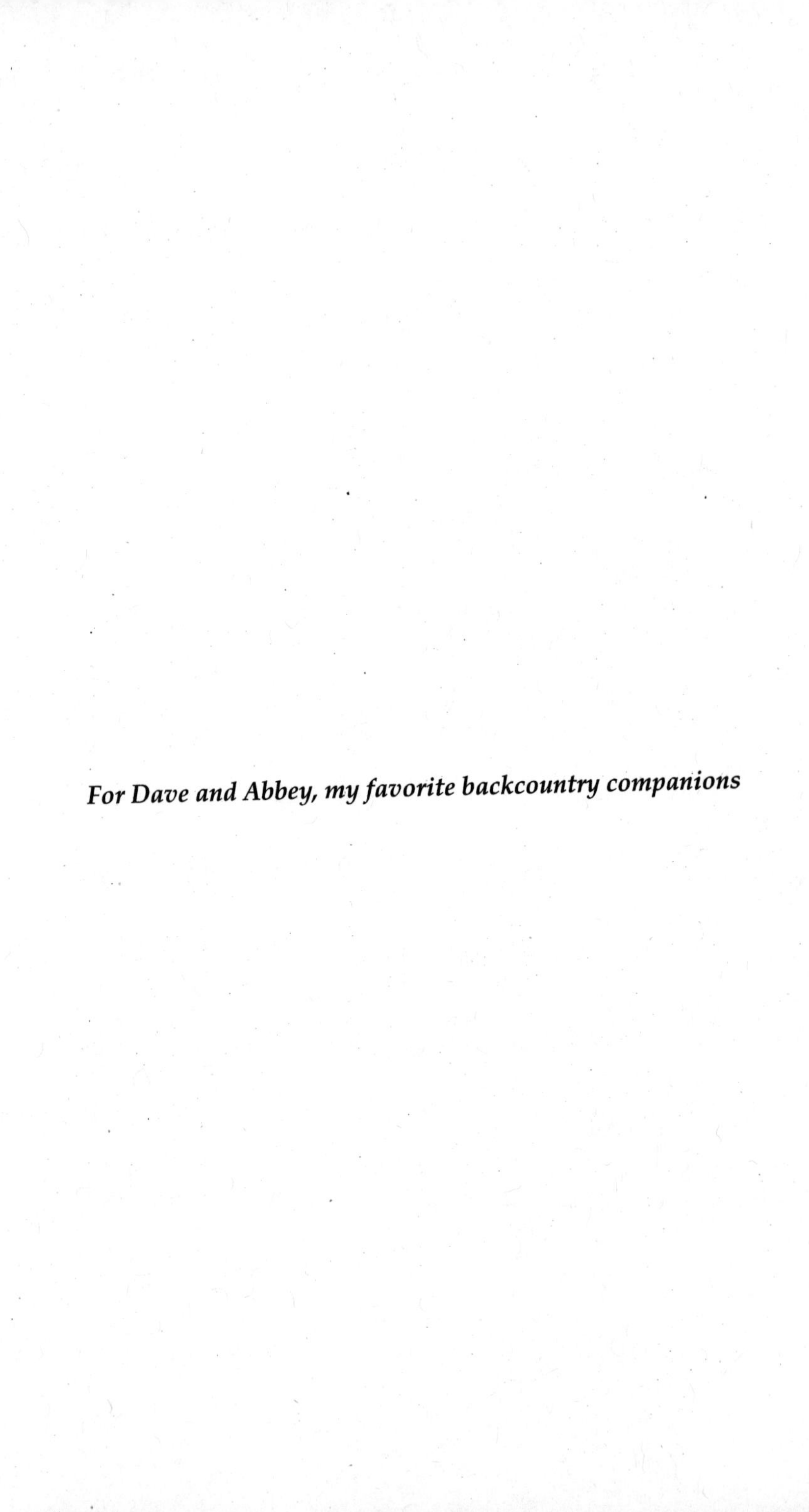

For Dave and Abbey, my favorite backcountry companions

Foreword

I first met Mary Howley Ryan when she enrolled in our graduate program in nutrition at the University of Utah. I soon came to realize that she was no ordinary nutrition graduate student. She had lived in a teepee and worked as a bartender before deciding to pursue a career in nutrition. Mary soon enthusiastically began to make the rounds of local grocery stores collecting unneeded food items for the homeless shelter in Salt Lake City in her old pickup truck and then began conducting cooking classes for the homeless on how to prepare sanitary and healthful meals to help prepare them for the day they would leave the shelter.

I had many discussions with Mary about another of her interests, wilderness nutrition. Mary was an avid backpacker and skier and wanted to apply her newly acquired dietetic skills to gain expertise in backcountry nutrition planning. Mary and I conducted a backcountry nutrition workshop for a Wilderness Medical Society meeting, and it was evident that she had the right stuff: the physicians loved her practical nutrition tips. As part of her graduate training, we arranged for her to visit Claudia Pearson at NOLS in Lander, Wyoming, where Mary helped evaluate some of the NOLS field menus. Mary loaded up her pickup with a laptop we loaned her, a long extension cord, and a tent, and spent the summer camped out in Claudia's backyard working on the NOLS rations.

While engaged in that summer of menu analysis, Mary and Claudia discussed preparing a small handbook on backcountry nutrition planning that could fit into a backpack and would weigh less than a bar of soap. Out of this discussion came the highly acclaimed 2002 NOLS publication, *NOLS Nutrition Field Guide*. We used this field guide as the text for our wilderness nutrition course offered at the University of Utah. It soon became evident that many of the readers of her nutrition field guide wanted even more of her practical and easy to understand nutrition advice. I encouraged Mary to write a full-length book on the topic. There were several good outdoor cookbooks on the market, but they did not delve into the nutrition behind their recipes to the extent that we would have liked, particularly for instructing our students on the "why" of nutrition rather than the just the "how."

The book she has written, *NOLS Backcountry Nutrition: Eating Beyond the Basics*, is remarkable from several aspects: it is very readable (doesn't read like a nutrition textbook!), contains sound nutrition advice and recommendations that Mary has tested herself during her backcountry excursions, and is a great how-to planning guide for the individual backpacker as well as the person in charge of planning the food for groups in the backcountry far from the closest grocery store. Her book fills a unique niche as a backcountry nutrition planner's guide. The chapters are interspersed with handy tips in the form of nutrition nuggets and pithy quotes that carry the reader from one topic to another. You certainly won't find this book boring, and you may want to carry it in your backpack, even if it does weigh more than a bar of soap!

—Dr. Wayne Askew, Director of the Division of Nutrition at the University of Utah

Acknowledgments

Claudia Pearson, the longtime rations department manager at NOLS Rocky Mountain, tops the list of people who motivated me to pursue this project, beginning with the first *NOLS Nutrition Field Guide* in 2002. Claudia has remained a source of positive energy and good ideas throughout this process, and her passion for making NOLS rations that support healthy, happy, and energetic backcountry travelers—without sacrificing taste and creativity—continues to inspire me as a nutrition educator and writer.

I would also like to thank Dr. Wayne Askew, Director of the Division of Nutrition at the University of Utah, for his continued encouragement and support of my nutrition endeavors. In addition to his expertise related to many backcountry nutrition topics, his enthusiasm for the subject and his sense of humor kept me in touch with the two things that helped me move forward and stay sane—thinking and laughing.

Dave, my husband and my biggest fan, has shared many insights and ideas about the reality of nutrition in a variety of backcountry situations, based on his experience as a mountain guide, avid climber, backcountry skier, and mountaineer. Dave's unending encouragement and creative suggestions—the Backcountry Nutrition Pinnacle and the field tips that I call "nutrition nuggets" were his ideas—kept me excited about this project.

I am also grateful to my family for their lifelong support of everything that I do. It was my mom who first introduced me to camping and taught me that improvisation in the kitchen is not only a necessity, but it also can produce creative and delicious results. My sister, Kelly, has been there to listen or make me laugh, depending on the day; and my brother, Joe, believed in me as a writer long before I did. Joe, whose favorite saying is "Camping is when the ice machine is on a different floor," is not much of a mentor regarding anything to do with the backcountry, but he is always there to encourage my writing. Then there is my dad; though no longer here to encourage me, he led me to my passion for this career path.

Although Mom first took me camping and taught me to cook, it was my friend Mary who introduced me to backpacking and showed me what is possible in a backcountry kitchen. I've had the good fortune to share backcountry meals and experiences with many great friends including Mary, Andrea, Martha, Andrew, Lizzie, Chris, and Norm—my expedition mates from NOLS ABW 2000—and also our fearless leaders Chris, Sarah, and Louie . . . I wish I had room to list them all.

Finally I would like to thank the staff at NOLS and Stackpole for giving me the opportunity to expand the original nutrition field guide to reach a broader audience with the message that food can enhance the backcountry experience. I am especially grateful to Joanne Kuntz, Book Publishing Coordinator at NOLS, who was a patient and thorough editor and did a great job coordinating feedback from various staff members at NOLS.

Introduction

So we find ourselves as a species almost back to where we started: anxious omnivores struggling once again to figure out what it is wise to eat.

—Michael Pollan, *The Omnivore's Dilemma*

At one time backcountry nutrition consisted of taking enough food and water for survival, making sure it didn't spoil, and planning for enough fuel to prepare it. While that is still a prevailing attitude towards nutrition for many weekend backcountry adventurers, those who choose to spend extended periods of time in the backcountry recognize the important role that food plays in going beyond the survival mode. Those who actually dare to enjoy their backcountry experience will appreciate this guide.

Food has always been an important part of the backcountry experience for the National Outdoor Leadership School (NOLS). The bulk rations system, combined with *NOLS Cookery,* encourages students to learn to fuel themselves throughout the day and cook creatively outdoors at mealtimes. After reviewing a study of the NOLS rations in 1999 and graduating from a twenty-eight-day NOLS Absaroka Backpacking course in 2000, I wrote the first *NOLS Nutrition Field Guide*. The initial guide provides an excellent start for NOLS students and instructors to learn how to put the rations together in the field for optimal nutrition and enjoyment. This subsequent book takes things a few steps further and provides valuable information that reaches beyond the NOLS community.

Designed in a simple and straightforward way to present practical, science-based nutritional information in order to prepare you for your backcountry experience, this is the book you read before you start meal planning for a trip. It helps explain what will give you energy, build strength, keep your immune system strong, and minimize cranky moments (at least the ones that are nutrition related). This isn't a cookbook, though you will find a couple of basic recipes for energy bars that can be made in or out of the field (see appendix A). For recipes and more specific help with menu planning, *NOLS Cookery* is an excellent companion to this field guide.

This book is divided into two sections. The first provides a foundation for understanding the basics of backcountry nutrition. The second shows you how to apply the building blocks to life in the backcountry. The second section also includes information about some nutritional tradeoffs that must be made in the backcountry, as well as which of these to take home and which are best left in the backcountry. Throughout this book you will find tips called "nutrition nuggets" to help you apply in the field what you learn from these pages; these tips are based on my experience, both as a dietitian and an accomplished backcountry cook. The appendices include more detailed information that can help you plan your backcountry menu or teach a basic nutrition lesson in the field.

Although you need information about the various nutrients, such as what they do, how much you need, and which ones should be your priority, this may not be what keeps you flipping pages at midnight. I have tried to include something for every backcountry enthusiast, from the student anticipating her first backpacking course to the experienced outdoor educator or guide.

There are now many outdoor education programs and adventure travel organizations that allow people of all ages to go into the backcountry for extended trips. This new incarnation of the 2002 *NOLS Nutrition Field Guide* continues the NOLS mission of being a leader in outdoor education—this time with respect to backcountry nutrition.

SECTION I BACKCOUNTRY NUTRITION BASICS

Eating is not merely a material pleasure. Eating well gives spectacular joy to life and contributes immensely to goodwill and happy companionship. It is of great importance to the morale.

—Elsa Schiaparelli, Parisan Sportswear Designer (1890–1973)

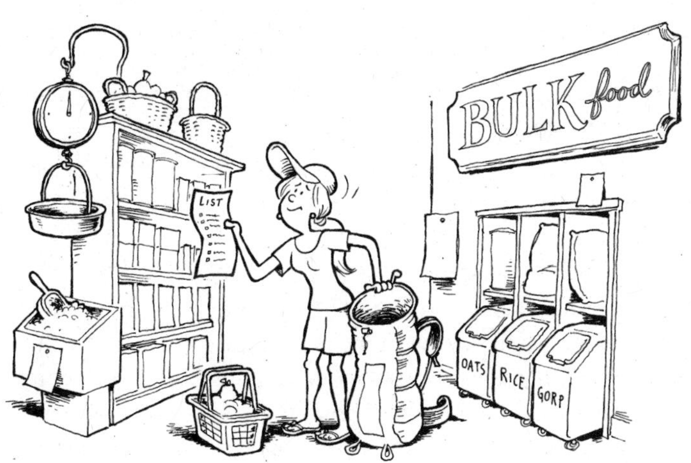

After more than twenty years of living in or close to mountain communities, surrounded by outdoor enthusiasts of all types and ages, I have observed that people seem more concerned about gear (including clothing) for their backcountry adventures than they are about food. While gear has certainly come a long way over the past few decades and can make backcountry travel lighter, easier, and potentially safer, there is no substitute for food and water for basic survival. Hence my mantra stemming from my NOLS internship several years ago: gear is good; food is better.

There are many factors that affect our food choices in the backcountry, and nutrition isn't typically at the top of the list. Of course, when we think of nutrition in its most basic forms—water and calories—we know that our survival, whether in the woods or our living room, depends upon nutrition. Our virtually unlimited access to food leaves us isolated from the "eat or die"mentality of our ancestors. Instead we tend to choose foods that taste good first. (And, for the record, taste *is* very important.) In fact, if your extended trip includes high-altitude conditions that can increase your need for food (while simultaneously decreasing your appetite), ensuring that you have food you want to eat because it tastes good is paramount to success in that environment.

In addition to taste there are other things to think about before you plan your backcountry menu, such as:

How much room will be in your pack?
How much weight will you be hauling, including gear?
How long will you be in the backcountry?
Where are you going (hot, cold, high-altitude, or remote locations or a foreign country)?
How much fuel and water can you access on the trail?
Who will be your traveling companions?

Once you figure out how these things affect your meal planning, then you can think about nutritional considerations for choosing specific foods.

Factors that Affect Food Choices in the Backcountry

Food preferences
Weight, perishability, taste, and texture of foods
Pack space
Length of trip or ration period
Availability of water and fuel for food preparation
Environmental conditions (heat, humidity, cold, altitude, etc.)
Individual and group experience with cooking and food preparation
Special dietary needs (food allergies, medical conditions, etc.)
Beliefs about food and nutrition

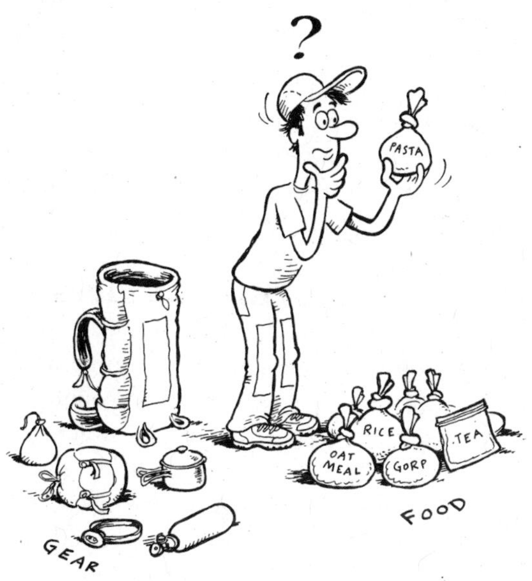

As the general introduction states, the goal of this book is to get beyond the basics and discover the many ways nutrition can actually help you enjoy your backcountry adventure. What you eat contributes to your health, strength, and energy levels, as well as your ability to think and focus; it also can affect your moods and how you relate to the other members of your group. The concept of expedition behavior (fondly referred to

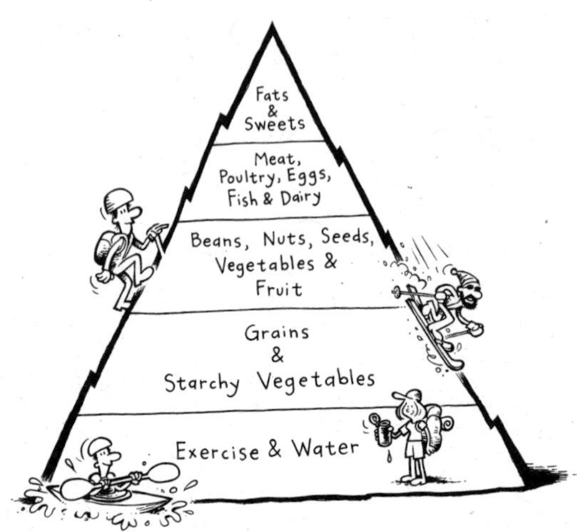

at NOLS as EB) means that fueling yourself properly is not only important for your individual well being, but it is part of what you do for the success of the entire expedition. Plainly spoken, eating well is "good EB."

BACKCOUNTRY NUTRITION PINNACLE

The general nutrition recommendations found in the USDA Food Pyramid must be adjusted in the backcountry to account for the limited available resources, such as water and fuel, for food preparation and cooking. Fresh foods are a luxury when pack space and weight must be shared with gear and clothing. Cost, perishability, length of the trip or ration period, and environmental conditions must also be considered for meal planning.

In light of these considerations, as well as the increased fluid needs and amount of physical activity involved in backcountry travel, the most recent edition of *NOLS Cookery* introduced a modified version of the food pyramid recommendations called the Backcountry Nutrition Pinnacle. (See appendix B for a breakdown of the food groups in the Pinnacle and recommendations for each.)

The Pinnacle adapts the USDA's general nutrition recommendations to the backcountry. There is an emphasis on water and additional carbohydrate foods to fuel exercise; and nuts, seeds, and beans (legumes) are included with fruits and vegetables since they contain many of the same nutrients. The first half of this book more fully explains the various nutrients you need in the backcountry, why you need them, how much you need, and where to find them in backcountry foods. Chapter 12 in the second half of this book highlights nutrition for the frontcountry, clarifying some of the nutritional tradeoffs made in the backcountry that are best left in the field.

A WELL-BALANCED BACKCOUNTRY MEAL

Aside from specific foods that contain important nutrients for backcountry travel, there are other important considerations such as when or how often you should eat. You may have all the right stuff nutritionally but not eat it when your body needs it most (or not eat it at all in the case of cook groups that return certain foods from the fields). If you are accustomed to regular, planned meal times, the idea that you need to eat when you are hungry in the backcountry throughout the day may be foreign to you. Or consider the situation where you are working really hard carrying a heavy pack uphill all day and you must learn to make yourself eat and drink even though you don't feel hungry or thirsty. These circumstances require you to ignore cultural beliefs and conventions, even some that are persistent nutritional myths, like all carbohydrate foods make you fat; or others that just aren't practical during backcountry travel, like a daily minimum of 7 to 9 servings of vegetables and fruit every day for good health. The backcountry presents many challenges, and a big one is the need to balance your nutritional needs with what is practical for your particular adventure.

CHAPTER 1 ENERGY: YOUR BACKCOUNTRY FUEL

If hunger makes you irritable, better eat and be pleasant.
—Sefer Hasidim, ancient Jewish doctrine

Never eat more than you can lift.
—Miss Piggy

When we talk about energy in relation to food, we are talking about calories. The word calorie is commonly used to refer to the amount of energy we get from our food. If you have studied science you may recall that a food calorie is technically a kilocalorie or a kcal of energy. A kcal is the amount of energy required to raise 1 kilogram of water 1 degree Celsius. For our purposes we will go with the common usage of the word calorie to refer to energy.

If we were concerned with survival only, this would be a very short book. First getting enough water and then enough calories from food to function in the backcountry would be the main message. If you ate and drank consistently, you would likely be fine. Of course, that gets back to the fact that you need to know enough to eat—not only when you are physically hungry—but also when you are too stressed, tired, or focused to experience hunger and thirst. Getting the right combination of protein, carbohydrates, fat, fiber, vitamins, and minerals is what allows you to stay healthy, build muscle, think clearly, and feel well, but in the end it is calories and water that keep you alive. There are many ways to estimate just how many calories you need to fuel various backcountry activities.

> ▶ **Exercise raises your body temperature, and higher body temperature decreases your appetite.**

ESTIMATING YOUR CALORIE NEEDS

There are several ways to estimate the amount of energy you need each day, and for most backcountry travelers it isn't practical or necessary to carry a calculator to figure it out (if you do choose to use a calculator, you are estimating based on formulas only). It is helpful to have a general idea about the number of calories you need for a strenuous day of backcountry travel, but it is even more important to know what that is in terms of food choices. If you have no idea what 3,000 calories a day is when applied to food, the numbers are meaningless. The following menu gives you a sample of a three-thousand-calorie day in the field, and there are other sample field menus in appendix F.

Menu for 3,000-calorie Day in the Field (not including water)

Food	*Amount*	*Calories*
Breakfast		
Instant oatmeal	2 packets	209
Raisins	1/4 cup	109
Walnut halves	1/4 cup	164
Powdered milk (cereal and extra for cocoa)	1/2 cup	122
Hot cocoa	1 packet	70
On the Trail (throughout the day)		
Yogurt covered peanuts	1/2 cup	460
Bagel (plain)	one (3″)	157
Cheddar cheese, sharp	2 oz.	240
Fig bar cookies	4	223
Soy nuts, salted	1 oz. (1/3 cup)	120
Clif Bar, Choc. Brownie	1	236
Tang, orange drink mix	2 Tbs.	92
Back at Camp		
Macaroni and cheese	2 cups	820
Sun-dried tomatoes	4 pieces	21
Herbal tea	12 oz.	3
Hot cocoa	1 packet	70
Totals		**3,115 calories**

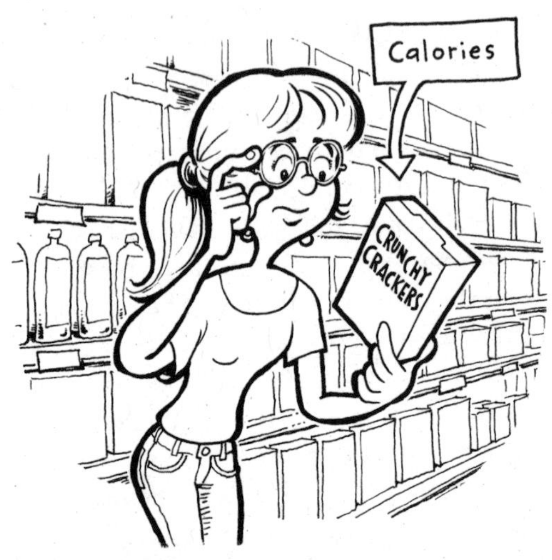

Appendix C contains a table with the nutritional breakdown of foods commonly issued for NOLS courses, many of which are common backcountry foods. You can use the table to help put together your own sample menu or to estimate how much energy (calories) you will get from these backcountry staples.

Based on the method you use for meal planning, you may estimate the number of calories you will need for your trip and divide it into ration periods if it is longer than a week. Next you must decide how to divide the calories into meals and snacks and make sure there is a good balance of carbohydrate, protein, and fat (ideally using foods that also have vitamins, minerals, and dietary fiber). For trips longer than a week to ten days, a bulk rationing system such as the one used by NOLS (see appendix C for an overview of the bulk rations system) allows greater flexibility and creativity than preplanned meals. Even if you use a combination of bulk items and preplanned meals, the NOLS system gives you an approximate idea of how many pounds of food per person is needed each day to get the calorie range you need. At NOLS the pounds per person per day varies for different types of trips (backpacking, climbing, boating, mountaineering, skiing, etc.).

There are several ways to estimate your calorie needs. Typically you begin with an equation that estimates your basic needs, and then you add calories for specific activities throughout the day. The most accurate way (and most laborious) is to begin by calculating your Resting Energy Expenditure (REE). This is the amount of energy it takes for everyday living such as breathing, thinking, heart beating, and producing hormones and antibodies. This is also known as basal metabolism and is basically all the functions your body performs whether you are on the couch or on the trail.

There are many factors that can influence your REE—caffeine intake or climatic conditions such as extreme temperatures and high altitude are some examples. Caffeine is a stimulant and two or three cups of regular coffee may increase REE as much as 10 to 12 percent. Sweating and shivering can dramatically increase REE, and high altitude exposure that makes breathing more difficult can also increase your basic calorie needs.

Estimation of the Daily Resting Energy Expenditure (REE)[1]

Age (years)	*Equation*
Males	
10 to 17	(17.5 × body weight*) + 651
18 to 29	(15.3 × body weight) + 679
30 to 60	(11.6 × body weight) + 879
Females	
10 to 17	(12.2 × body weight*) + 746
18 to 29	(14.7 × body weight) + 496
30 to 60	(8.7 × body weight) + 829

*Weight in kilograms (kg) (kg = pounds divided by 2.2; e.g. 150 lbs. ÷ 2.2 = 68 kg)

[1]REE does not include calories needed for physical activity; it is the baseline of calories used for basic functions.

Technically, the next part of your total daily needs includes the Thermic Effect of Food (TEF) or the amount of energy you need to digest food assuming you eat a mixed diet of carbohydrates, proteins, and fats. This is usually about 5 to 10 percent of your total daily energy expenditure.

Lastly, you add the Thermic Effect of Exercise (TEE), which is based on what you do for the day. This will vary a lot depending on your backcountry day. So a rest day when you lounge around camp or maybe learn to fish or identify wild

> **▶ You may eat more on a rest day than you think you need in response to your high level of activity on other days. Relax—this is normal.**

edibles will require less energy (calories/food) than a long day of hiking with a fifty-pound pack. Hiking uphill or traversing through snow will require more calories than belaying your climbing partner, floating a stretch of flat water, or skiing downhill.

The reality is, if you use the REE and the TEE, you will have a close enough estimate to plan your menu. It is good for you to realize, however, that digestion does burn some calories and generates heat. This is important in cold environments when you need to stay warm; not only do you need calories to let you shiver (one way we generate heat for warmth), but the very act of eating and digesting creates some heat.

PUTTING IT ALL TOGETHER

Now you have an estimate of your basic needs based on your age and body weight (from the REE table on the previous page), before you add any physical activity (exercise or camp

Calories Used Per Hour for Various Activities

Activity Level	*Activity*	*Calories Used Per Hour*
Very Light	Seated and standing activities (cooking, playing cards)	80 to 100
Light	Walking on level surface at 2.5 to 3 mph, sailing, golf, etc.	110 to 160
Moderate	Walking 3.5 to 4 mph, carrying a load, cycling, skiing, tennis, dancing, etc.	170 to 240
Heavy	Walking with a load uphill, heavy manual digging, climbing, football, soccer, etc.	250 to 350
Very Heavy	Professional athletic training	350+

Sources: The National Research Council, "Recommended Dietary Allowances" (Washington, D.C.: National Academy Press, 1989). "Food and Your Weight," *House and Garden Bulletin*, No. 74 (Washington, D.C.: U.S. Department of Agriculture).

chores). You can use the tables on pages 10 and 11 to estimate how many calories per hour you need for a general activity level. For example, to estimate your calorie needs for a mellow, relatively inactive, rest day, calculate your REE and then add the calories per hour based on very light or light activities.

Alternately, forget the REE, and multiply your weight by the range of calories per pound for a less active activity level, and you will have a range for a less active day. The activity categories in the following table are a quick way to estimate daily calorie needs. They are suggested activities and calorie requirements that may compare to activities of backcountry travel,

Calories Used Per Day Based on Weight

Less Active

(Rest day, easy camp chores, recovery day, etc.)

Body weight (lbs.) × (both) 13.5 to 15 calories per pound = range of calories used per day

Example: 130 lbs. × (both) 14 to 15 = 1,820 to 1,950 calories/day

Moderately Active

(45 to 60 minutes of purposeful moderate intensity exercise; easy day hiking, skiing, or climbing with little or no extra weight from a pack)

Body weight (lbs.) × (both) 16 to 20 calories per pound = range of calories used per day

Example: 130 lbs. × (both)16 to 20 = 2,080 to 2,600 calories per day

Very Active

(60 to 120 minutes of purposeful moderate exercise: hiking, climbing, or skiing that involves hills and carrying a pack)

Body weight (lbs.) × (both) 21 to 25 calories per pound = range of calories used per day

Example: 130 lbs. × (both) 21 to 25 = 2,730 to 3,250 calories per day

Extremely Active

(Training for an ultra-endurance event: long, strenuous day of hiking, skiing, or climbing with heavy pack)

Body weight (lbs.) × (both) 25 to 30 calories per pound = range of calories used per day

Example: 130 lbs. × (both) 25 to 30 = 3,250 to 3,900 calories per day

Endurance Sports Nutrition, Susan Eberle

Too Many Calories?

Remember that all of these calculations for estimating your calorie needs are just that, estimates. Also, many of the estimates are based on weight. The weight you carry—whether it is your own body fat, a heavy backpack, heavy gear and clothing for a winter expedition, or hauling a sled with provisions—is all weight that contributes to your calorie needs.

Some backcountry enthusiasts who have adopted the "light and fast" trend argue that an individual needs less food than many of these calculations suggest. If you lighten your load (either by losing body weight or by carrying lighter gear), you may need fewer calories, unless you significantly increase your exercise intensity. If you are an experienced backcountry traveler, you have probably figured out what you need in terms of calories, and it may differ from what you calculate here.

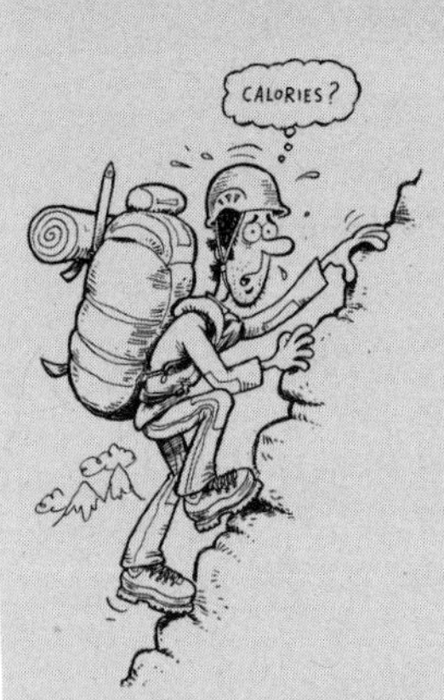

However, the main tenet of this book is to go beyond survival to fully enjoy your backcountry experience. One bad storm in the backcountry can drastically increase your calorie needs, and if you are too close to the wire in terms of food supplies, you may be forced into a food shortage. Forced fasting, particularly in a bad weather situation, can be dangerous. Not fueling properly can affect your ability to think clearly and make good decisions. If you are not highly experienced in the type of backcountry trip you are planning, these calculations can help you estimate your calorie needs, and you can view any excess calories you take along as a margin of safety.

though they are just estimates. Also, once your body adjusts to the routine of long days of backcountry exercise, the number of calories burned for the same activity may decrease.

The energy you need for camp chores will vary greatly depending on many factors. The season (winter or summer), the environment (hot, cold, or high altitude), how many of you there are to divide the work, how close you are to a water source, and the type of trip you are doing (mountaineering, boating, backpacking, skiing, etc.) will all affect how much

► You may need to schedule food and water breaks during strenuous exercise or in hot or high-altitude climates.

Calories Burned in the Field

Activity	*Amount of time*	*Calories burned for a 130-lb. adult*	*Calories burned for a 180-lb. adult*
Camping (basic activities)	4 hours	590	816
Fishing (from bank, walking)	2 hours	472	653
Hiking (general)	5 hours	1,769	2,449
Hill climb (with a 42+-lb. pack)	5 hours	2,654	3,674
Hunting (general)	5 hours	1,474	2,041
Rock climbing (uphill)	3 hours	1,946	2,694
Skiing (2.5 mph, cross country with no pack)	5 hours	2,064	2,858
Snow mountaineering	5 hours	4,865	6,736
Snowshoeing	2 hours	943	1,306
Whitewater canoeing, kayaking, or rafting	5 hours	1,474	2,041

www.caloriesperhour.com

> ► **There is no magic in dehydrated, packaged meals. They are lightweight and often more expensive than other packaged foods. If you decide to use these, try them first to make sure you like them, you can digest them well, and that the serving sizes are appropriate for you (often they claim to make two servings but one hungry mountaineer can eat the whole package, or more!). When using dehydrated meals, hydrate halfway with boiled water, cover, and steep for 5–10 minutes. Finish hydrating with additional boiled water so it is hot when served.**

energy you expend. Also, body weight affects the calories that you burn. If you weigh 180 pounds, you will burn more calories camping than if you weigh 130 pounds. The point here is that basic camping activities burn calories too, including all of the various things that this entails, such as hauling water, putting up tents, cooking, hanging food to protect it from critters, and finding the best spot when Mother Nature calls. The calculations in the previous table use body weight and the calories burned for specific activities based on the activity calculator found at www.caloriesperhour.com. However, they are only estimates.

Throughout this book, you will be reminded that if you get enough calories (energy) from a variety of foods in order to fuel your backcountry activities, you will have the best chance of meeting your nutritional needs in the field. See appendix D for a full explanation of how to estimate calorie needs for a complete day with a variety of activities. The chapters that follow will discuss how to fine-tune your backcountry diet to make sure that your food delivers more than merely calories. Once again: enough water and calories means survival; enough of everything else enhances your backcountry experience.

NOLS Going Light

During the forty-plus years that NOLS has been taking people into the backcountry, there have been many changes with respect to gear, clothing, and food. In keeping with these changes NOLS is currently aiming to decrease the pack weight of its courses to benefit the health and well-being of students and staff. In considering how to take less weight into the field, however, NOLS must also maintain the ability to teach a variety of skills, be prepared for the environment (changing weather conditions or medical emergencies), adequately hydrate, and eat well.

Because of the high calorie needs during many of the backpacking and mountaineering courses, the issue of reducing the rations poses a challenge. Cooking and eating in the backcountry is a big part of the NOLS experience, so lightening the load must be done in a way that still allows students and instructors to continue to eat well.

A related trend that has caught the school's attention is characterized as "go light." In order to begin introducing a few specialized "lightweight" backpacking courses each year, NOLS has partnered with both Go Lite and Backpacking Light; Go Lite is a company that specializes in making light backcountry gear and clothing, and Backpacking Light is an online magazine that helps plan and implement the fast-and-light approach to backcountry travel. The idea is to incorporate the lightest gear and clothing appropriate for the trip (considering terrain, climate, and length of time in the field) and still teach the skills and leadership necessary to thrive in the backcountry. However, going light has also meant reevaluating food rations.

The goal of special rations for light courses is to concentrate calories and minimize packaging. Special lightweight alcohol stoves require minimal cooking time, so quick-cooking thin or small pastas or foods that do not require any cooking, such as jerky and pouches of tuna, are part of these rations. Special high-calorie sauces are added to the quick-cooking or instant grains for dinners that meet the need for nutrition, taste, and, of course, low weight (along with minimal pack space).

Because the amount of lightweight rations looks sparse compared to more standard rations, and the necessary calories and nutrients are condensed into less food, this approach does require buy-in from participants. But, so far, the courses have been very well received, including the special food rations.

CHAPTER 2

WATER: YOU CAN'T LIVE WITHOUT IT

Drinking a daily cup of tea will surely starve the apothecary.
—Chinese Proverb

Water is, without a doubt, the most important nutrient in the backcountry. If forced to, humans can survive weeks without food but only days without water (and even less if the dehydration involves rapid water loss). Aside from the catastrophic result of no water, without enough fluid you cannot perform your best. About half to three-quarters of your body weight is water, and 70 to 75 percent of your muscles are water. So even though water does not directly provide you with energy (like calories do), all of the cells in your body need fluid to work properly. You need water to lubricate your joints, cushion your organs and tissues, and produce saliva and gastric juices to digest your food. Not getting enough water in the field can make you feel tired, lethargic, and crabby; affect how well your muscles work; and cause headaches and gastrointestinal problems (cramps, constipation, bloating, and stomach pain). Water is also needed to transport nutrients throughout your body, to get rid of metabolic waste products, and to regulate your body temperature.

HOW MUCH WATER DO YOU NEED?

Similar to calories, the amount of water you need varies with physical activity and environmental conditions. Extreme heat or cold, humidity or dryness, and high altitude all increase your

Water Disinfection

There are many backcountry travelers who cannot let go of the romanticized vision of drinking pure, clean water from a backcountry stream. As lovely as this fantasy is, the reality is that much of our backcountry water may be contaminated with bacteria, viruses, and protozoa, no matter how clean it looks.

According to the U.S. Environmental Protection Agency (EPA), *Giardia lamblia* and *Cryptosporidium* are the two microorganisms frequently found in rivers and lakes. Cloudy water should ideally be filtered through a clean cloth (a bandana works in a pinch), or allow the debris to settle and pour off the clear water to boil. According to the Wilderness Medicine Institute of NOLS, bringing water to a rolling boil is enough to disinfect water at any altitude.

Obviously, boiling is not the best option during the day when you need water on the trail. The good news is there are many systems available to disinfect backcountry water, ranging from the inexpensive, lightweight, and easy-to-use iodine or chlorine-based tablets, to a variety of high-tech filters. There are also several slick new systems based on technology tested in the military that use a battery-charged electric brine solution and others that use ultraviolet light as a disinfectant. According to the EPA, both iodine and chlorine are more effective in warm water than cold water and are more effective in protecting against *Giardia* than the more resistant microorganisms like *Cryptosporidium.* Regardless of your threshold for taste (some cannot tolerate the taste of iodine) and your budget, there are no excuses for not having some form of water disinfection in the backcountry.

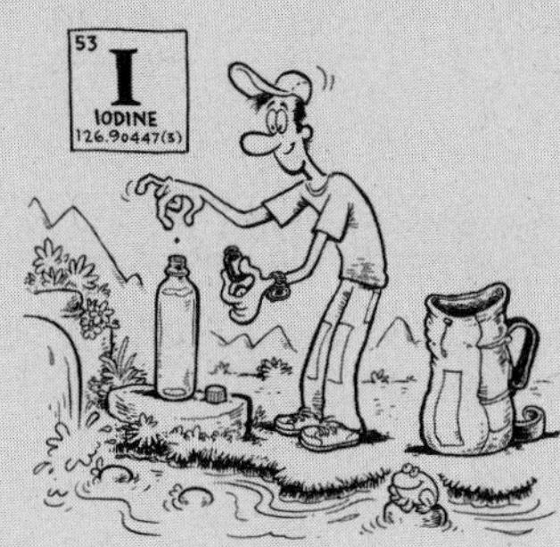

water needs. In general, the amount of fluid you need relates to the amount of your food and fluid intake versus what you lose through sweat, urine, feces, breathing, and skin—this is called water balance. An easy way to estimate your basic fluid needs is to think in terms of your intake of calories and then add more for exercise and environmental conditions accordingly (high altitude, extreme heat, cold, etc.). If you regularly eat 2,000 calories per day, you need 2 to 3 quarts of water per day. In the backcountry, when you are using anywhere from 3,000 to 5,000 calories

Tips for Bottles and Bladders

- Use water bottles for drink mix, not your hydration pack. It is too difficult to clean water bladders and tubes well in the backcountry to prevent bacterial growth.
- For long trips or locations where water sources are not too close to camp, dromedaries are a great way to store more water at camp than you can (or want to) carry.
- Use Teflon tape to cover the threads of your water bottle so it doesn't leak. (This is important if you decide to put a water bottle filled with hot water at the bottom of your sleeping bag on a winter trip to warm your feet!)
- Protect your hydration pack bladder from punctures, and carry a patch kit (as well as a backup water bottle).

► **Each group member needs some form of water treatment. If you decide to bring one filter for a group, make sure that everyone who is not carrying the filter has iodine tablets or some other solution for emergency use.**

per day, you will need 3 to 6 quarts of water a day and possibly more with excessive water losses from sweat and diarrhea, or if you are recovering from an illness (see chapter 8 for more info about backcountry illnesses).

The sports nutrition mantra for hydration is "drink early and drink often" when exercising. You don't typically get thirsty until you have lost 1.5 to 2 liters of water, or roughly 2 percent of your body weight, in sweat (that is three pounds of body weight for a 150-pound person). Sweat is the way your body keeps cool, and when you exercise in the backcountry, there are several situations when you don't know how much fluid you are losing. A very dry or windy day means sweat can evaporate before you feel it. If you are carrying a heavy pack or bundled up in winter garb, you may not realize how much sweat you produce until you take off your pack or clothing layers once you've stopped moving.

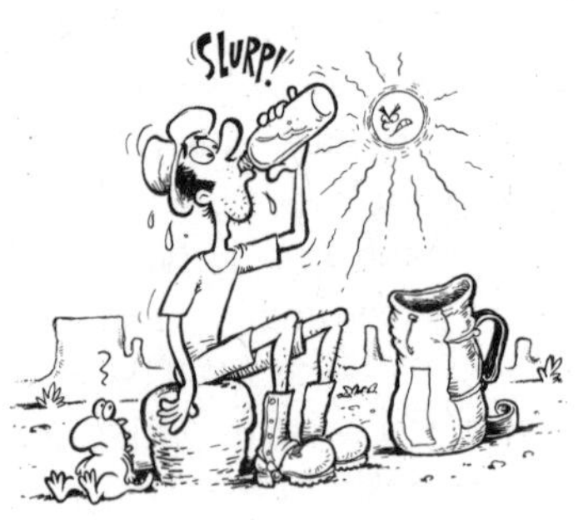

The rate of sweating also varies among individuals. Some are more prone to dehydration than others, so this is something to watch for in the field. The maximal sweat rate for a trained athlete is roughly 2 to 3 liters per hour. Two liters of sweat equals 4.4 pounds. A 150-pound runner can lose 3 percent of body weight in one hour ($4.4/150 = 0.03 \times 100 = 3\%$). Even if you are not a trained athlete, losing sweat at a high rate per hour over the course of a strenuous day of backpacking, and especially in a hot environment, you can lose a significant amount of water.

Since individuals sweat at different rates, many sports nutritionists recommend weighing yourself before and after a workout to figure out how much water you lose. Great idea—unless you are in the backcountry, where the more general way to tell if you are well hydrated is to make sure you are urinating regularly and the color is like straw. The caveats here are, if you are going out into the cold or adjusting to high altitude, you may urinate more frequently in response to those conditions (this is called diuresis) and actually need to drink more fluid even if you are urinating a lot. Also, if you are taking a vitamin supplement (including Emergen-C packets), certain vitamins give urine a bright yellow color, so color is a less accurate measure of how well hydrated you are. Basically, you don't want a trickle of dark urine or

did you know ?

We depend upon both *food* and *fluid* intake to adequately hydrate.

Food contains water. This is obvious in the case of many fruits and vegetables that are 60 to 90 percent water, and less obvious with drier foods such as bread, which is 36 percent water. In the backcountry we try to take dried foods to keep our pack weight down; then we add the water back when we prepare the food. Either way, we rely on the water content of food.

Food also provides water when it is used for energy. For example, 350 grams of carbohydrates contributes one liter of water for body functions. This includes both the water contained in the carbohydrate food and the water produced from metabolizing the food.

Food is also an important source of electrolytes, (sodium, potassium, and chloride) that are needed to balance body water properly.

The water we get from food does not replace the need to drink fluids; however, not eating properly in the field may contribute to dehydration.

Risk Factors for Dehydration

Extreme heat, cold, humidity
High altitude
High protein diet
High sodium diet
Vomiting, diarrhea
Infection, fever
Inadequate fluid intake
Medications
Laxatives
Diuretics (may include caffeine, varies according to use)

did you know ?

In heat, up to **3 liters of fluid may be lost per hour through sweat!** This is approximately 50 ml per minute, and only 20 to 30 ml of fluid per minute may be absorbed from the intestines. This means you cannot absorb fluid fast enough to replace the fluid you lose exercising in hot environments. Remember to drink before, during, and after physical activity in the heat to keep up with your fluid needs.

hours without producing any. Constipation, bloating, and stomach or muscle cramps are other signs that you may not be getting enough fluid.

If you know you sweat a lot and you are exercising for more than three hours in the heat, you should plan to drink the higher end of the recommendations and make sure that you are eating salty foods at meals and snacks. Also, if you are not eating regularly throughout the day, you may want to combine plain water with some kind of drink mix that has salt and ideally some potassium (see information about hyponatremia at the end of this chapter). If you are eating regularly at and between meals, plain water is probably fine unless you know you are losing excessive fluid due to any of the reasons mentioned above.

Symptoms of Dehydration

Weakness
Headache
Fatigue
Lethargy
Constipation
Mental confusion
Increased heart rate
Decreased urine output
Dark-colored urine output

Terms Related to Hydration

Water balance: balance of water intake and excretion that keeps body water content constant.

Fluid and electrolyte balance: maintenance of proper amounts and types of fluids and minerals in body compartments.

Dehydration: loss of body water.

ELECTROLYTES

Sports drinks, gels, and bars often tout their electrolyte content as a plus for fueling exercise. An electrolyte is a substance that conducts electric current in solution, and water needs the help of these compounds to perform its various functions in the body. Your body uses the electrolytes—sodium, potassium, magnesium, calcium, chloride, bicarbonate, and sulfate—to conduct nerve impulses and activate various enzymes. You can have enough fluid on board, but if it isn't in the right places on a cellular level, you're in trouble. This can happen if you drink an excessively sweet beverage while exercising and your intestines draw water out of the cells to help your body absorb the fluid. This makes the cells and tissues dehydrated even though there is additional fluid coming in. (Note that sports drinks formulated to be consumed during exercise may taste sweet to some people but generally have the proper amount and types of sugar.)

Electrolytes are found in many popular backcountry foods. Sodium is the main electrolyte lost in sweat, and salt is made up of sodium and chloride (40 percent of salt is sodium). Nearly all packaged, canned, and processed foods are high in salt. Although this can be a problem in the frontcountry (particularly for people with high blood pressure or who are at risk for heart disease and stroke), in the backcountry it is a plus. Adding salt to a beverage helps your body hold onto the fluid more easily. This

► Ramen is a great source of sodium (salt), but due to concerns about salt in the general population, there are now different amounts of sodium in different types of ramen. Look for the higher sodium version to take into the backcountry.

Sodium Content of Popular Backcountry Foods

Foods and Beverages	***Serving Size***	***Amount of Sodium (mg)***
Powerbar	1	95 to 125
Triple Threat Powerbar	1	210
Clif Bar	1	150 to 210
Luna Bar	1	50
Larabar	1	0
Gu (sports gel)	1 pkg.	35 to 50
Gatorade	pkg. for 1 qt.	400
Gookinaid Hydralite	pkg. for 1 qt.	256
Bread	1 slice	130
Cheese	1 oz.	445
String cheese	1	200
Jerky	1 oz.	460+
Trail mix	1 oz.	14
Peanut butter	2 tbs.	120
Mixed nuts (salted, roasted)	1 oz.	55
Pretzels (large)	1	210
Triscuit crackers	6	180
Chex mix	$^{2}/_{3}$ cup	370
Hot cocoa	1 pkt.	180
Ramen Noodles + flavor pkt.	$^{1}/_{2}$ pkg.	600 to 900
Lunch meat	1 oz.	450
Mustard	1 tbs.	195

Note: Salt is 40% sodium and 60% chloride; 1 tsp. of salt = 5 grams NaCl = 2 grams sodium (2,000 mg).

Good Backcountry Sources of Potassium

- Dried apricots
- Bananas
- Chili peppers
- Chocolate
- Dates
- Dried beans and peas
- Figs
- Molasses
- Nuts and seeds
- Oranges
- Peanut butter
- Potatoes (baked, boiled, or mashed)
- Prunes (dried plums)
- Sports drinks
- Sweet potatoes (dehydrated)
- Tomato sauce/powder
- Tomato paste

may be why sports drinks taste better when used during exercise when your body needs that extra salt.

> ► Seaweed is a great source of sodium and other important minerals. It is also lightweight and easy to pack. Break it up and add it to soup or make a salty broth to replenish electrolytes at the end of the day.

When you exercise in the heat, you can lose 1,000 milligrams of sodium for every two pounds of sweat loss (and you can lose up to 2 to 3 liters in sweat per hour, particularly once you are fit and acclimated). This translates to a lot of sodium. One teaspoon of table salt (sodium chloride) contains roughly 2,400 milligrams of sodium. One salt tablet (500 to 875 milligrams of salt or NaCl) contains somewhere between 200 to 350 milligrams of sodium, and as you can see in the previous table, it is not difficult to get this much sodium from foods. While athletes competing in hot, humid environments for more than three hours may still be encouraged to use salt tablets, the average backcountry traveler, eating and drinking throughout the day, will get plenty of sodium (and other needed electrolytes) from foods. It is also helpful to know that if you are traveling in a hot environment, part of your body's adaptation to that climate is an increased sweat rate to cool your body, along with the ability to hold onto sodium to decrease the loss of this important electrolyte through sweat.

> ► Dried mushrooms are an excellent source of potassium and are great in backcountry soups and pasta meals (they also provide selenium, copper, B vitamins, and some protein; and some varieties have phytonutrients with anticancer properties).

SEX, AGE, AND FITNESS AFFECT WATER NEEDS

You may be familiar with the saying "muscle weighs more than fat." This is because muscle contains glycogen, the storage form of carbohydrates that your body uses for fuel, and muscle glycogen is stored with water. In fact, every gram of glycogen has roughly 3 grams of water along with it. As you burn through your glycogen stores, to fuel your activity, you release this water for your body to use. So the more muscle you have, the more water you can store.

This phenomenon has implications for sex, age, and fitness differences in terms of how often you need to drink. If you are a female, a teen, or a young adult with less muscle mass than your male or bigger (more muscle mass) expedition mates, you will need to drink (and eat) more often than they do. If you are more fit than other members of your group (assuming that you have more muscle mass), you may need to drink less often (unless you happen to sweat more). If you have more body fat and are less fit, your tolerance to heat will also be lower than those with more lean mass and better fitness.

> did you know?
>
> **Dehydration is cumulative.** If you end the day slightly dehydrated, you begin the next day dehydrated and will need more fluid than the day before to bring things into balance.

AT THE END OF THE DAY

It can take twenty-four hours or more to completely rehydrate after a long day in the field. This means it is important to drink throughout the day and then make an extra effort to drink throughout the evening to help you get ready to start the next day feeling well. One challenge related to hydration is that water is a diuretic. If you drink too much water at one time in an attempt to "catch up" with your fluid needs, your body cannot absorb the water fast enough and you will eliminate it. The best plan for hydration is to sip water throughout the day, allowing your body to maximize absorption, rather than to chug large amounts of water at the end of the day.

Even if you are sipping fluids throughout the day, however, the hydration process doesn't end with your day's activity. It is difficult (and possibly impractical) in many backcountry situations to drink enough during the day. Plus there is the cumulative aspect of dehydration; so even if you are well-hydrated, drinking 3 liters of water one day, there is no guarantee that 3 liters will be enough every day. Plan to drink at least .5 liter of water or another beverage right when you get to camp, and then plan to drink 2 liters or more throughout the evening depending on such things as how much you drank during the day, heat, humidity, cold, and altitude.

The NOLS tradition of hot drinks in the evenings is one many backcountry users enjoy and certainly contributes to hydration but really is not the best way to hydrate. If you cool the hot tea, cocoa, or cider to more of a warm temperature, you will drink more of it and it can be part of your evening rehydrating regimen. If you prefer to sip a hot beverage, definitely more appealing on an evening spent winter camping or at high altitude anytime of year, aim to drink your 2 liters (or more) before the leisurely sipping begins.

Commonly Asked Hydration Questions

Q: Shouldn't we be drinking a sports drink that contains electrolytes in the backcountry?

A: Sports drinks are formulated with carbohydrate (sugar) to keep glycogen stores topped off in working muscles and to maintain blood sugar levels. They also contain salt to replace sodium losses that occur in sweat during exercise, and many also have a small amount of potassium, another electrolyte lost in sweat. The drink mixes provided by NOLS are similar in carbohydrate composition to popular sports drinks (less than 10 percent carbohydrate) with the added bonus of vitamin C. Tang orange-flavored drink mix is available in grocery stores and is similar to the NOLS mixes but with less vitamin C. The mixes do not have as much sodium as many sports drinks (20 grams compared to 100 grams); however, eating a combination of meals and snacks throughout the day usually provides enough salt and other minerals so that plain water is sufficient for hydration.

If you are in a very hot or cold environment or know you sweat heavily, it is a good idea to add an occasional bottle of drink mix in place of plain water. There is no magic in sports drinks, however; in fact, in a pinch, just adding some salt and sugar to plain water can be an electrolyte replacement drink. For replenishing electrolytes without an Oral Rehydrating Solution (ORS), the World Health Organization recommends mixing 6 teaspoons of sugar, 1 teaspoon of salt, and 1 liter of safe (treated) water.

Q: Are muscle cramps caused by dehydration?

A: Muscle cramps may be due to several factors, including inadequate water intake.

In addition, electrolyte imbalance and a lack of potassium, sodium, and calcium have all been suspected of playing a role in muscle cramping. Calcium is an unlikely culprit given the fact that we store calcium in our bones and may access that as needed. If a loss of appetite for any reason has led to a decreased food intake, potassium or sodium may be involved. Generally, the food in NOLS rations and other common backcountry foods contain plenty of both of these electrolytes (see the Sodium Content of Popular Backcountry Foods and Good Backcountry Sources of Potassium tables in this chapter), so if you are eating trail foods and regular meals, a deficiency of these nutrients should not be a problem. However, there may be no nutritional role whatsoever; stretching and proper training are believed to be important for those predisposed to muscle cramping.

Q: Is room-temperature water more easily absorbed than cold water?
A: There is some research to show that during exercise cold water is actually absorbed faster than room-temperature water, but it isn't clear that the difference is significant. Cold water is more palatable in warm or hot environments, a factor that may encourage you to drink more fluid. Cold liquids also may assist with cooling core body temperature, in addition to providing water for sweat. If you are traveling in the winter, or even on a cold day in the summer, and you are chilled, cold water is not the best option because it does have the core cooling effect. Hot or warm liquids are a better choice in these situations and are probably the most appealing options anyway.

TOO MUCH OF A GOOD THING

While dehydration definitely has a negative affect on exercise performance, health, and sense of well-being, what is less clear, particularly among recreational athletes, is "how much water is too much?" Excessive hydration, especially combined with excessive sodium losses due to sweat, can result in a life threatening condition called hyponatremia. Although this is not a common occurrence in the backcountry apart from adventure and ultra-endurance competitions, there has been more discussion about it lately, and this condition has potentially serious consequences, especially for women.

WHAT IS HYPONATREMIA?

Hyponatremia is basically abnormally low blood sodium levels due to a fluid-electrolyte imbalance. Normal blood sodium concentrations are 136 to 142 mmol/liter (mmol is the abbreviation for millimole, a unit of measure) and hyponatremia occurs when levels drop below 135 mmol/liter. This reduction in blood sodium causes brain swelling that can lead to a number of serious neurological responses. There is a progression of symptoms that begin as blood sodium levels drop. Initial symptoms may include bloating and mild nausea, followed by throbbing headaches, vomiting, wheezy breathing, swollen hands and feet, restlessness, unusual fatigue, confusion, and disorientation. When levels drop further, seizure, respiratory arrest, coma, permanent brain damage, and death may occur.

WHO IS AT RISK?

There are several factors that increase the risk of developing hyponatremia. The biggest factor seems to be drinking too much water before and during prolonged exercise in warm climates. While marathon runners and Ironman-distance triathletes have made hyponatremia news headlines, this problem is also seen among other groups, such as military personnel and hikers in the Grand Canyon, and mountain guides in the Tetons have noted several cases among clients in recent years.

While adequate hydration in each of these situations remains an important goal for health and performance, an awareness that we can get too much water seems increasingly important. Currently there is an abundance of gear related to helping us hydrate more easily and efficiently. Many health-conscious athletes also avoid excess dietary sodium to treat or prevent high blood pressure.

There are also many medications, both prescription and over-the-counter (OTC), as well as illicit drugs, that may make individuals more susceptible to hyponatremia. NSAIDs (non-steroidal anti-inflammatory drugs) such as ibuprofen (Motrin, Advil, etc.) are commonly used OTC medications that can compromise kidney function during exercise, increasing the risk of hyponatremia. Prescription medications for blood pressure, depression, diabetes, cancer, Alzheimer's, and many other diseases and conditions can also cause problems. Opiates and the drug commonly known as ecstasy are illicit drugs that may lead to serious sodium imbalances.

CONSIDERATIONS FOR WOMEN

An awareness of hyponatremia is particularly important for women. Several studies report a higher number of female athletes who develop hyponatremia, yet most researchers believe that the reasons for these findings have more to do with habits than sex. Females tend to be more conscientious about hydrating than their male counterparts and perhaps get a bit carried away. However, the consequences of hyponatremia may be more serious for women than for men. Estrogen affects the enzymes that move potassium out of the brain. This potassium shift is an important response to the brain swelling that occurs with the abnormal loss of sodium. According to the Gatorade Sports Science Institute (GSSI), "young women in particular, who have higher levels of estrogen are twenty-five times more likely to die or have permanent brain damage following post-operative hyponatremic brain swelling compared to men or postmenopausal women, who have relatively low levels of estrogen."

Another issue for many women is their small body size. In fact, according to the GSSI, "although larger athletes are not immune to hyponatremia, small, slow athletes who sweat a lot, excrete a salty sweat, and are overzealous in their drinking habits are theoretically at greater risk." The reasoning here is that it takes less fluid to dilute the blood in a small body, slower athletes have more time to consume excessive fluids, and individuals vary in the amount of sodium (salt contains 40 percent sodium, 60 percent chloride) in their sweat.

For athletes who exercise in warm climates, acclimatization is also important. When our bodies adjust to a warm climate, our sweat glands conserve sodium, thereby reducing the risk of developing hyponatremia. There are some athletes, however, even very fit athletes, that just sweat more than average.

HOW MUCH WATER IS TOO MUCH?

Some of the more publicized cases of hyponatremia illustrate the extremes. One individual consumed 3 liters of water per hour in an attempt to throw off a pending drug test. Soldiers training in extreme conditions consumed 9 to 20 liters of water over a few hours, and a female marathon runner drank 10 liters of fluid the night before a race. While studies show that adults drinking roughly 1.5 liters of water per hour over 2 to 3 hours reduced their blood levels of sodium, most adults can handle occasional imbalances by excreting the excess fluid as urine.

There is no specific amount of water that is appropriate for everyone, so it is important to be aware of the factors that contribute to hyponatremia, the early warning signs that you may have overdone it with water intake, and what to do to address the situation. Including a mix of water and beverages (or foods) that include sodium during prolonged exercise can usually correct an electrolyte imbalance and prevent hyponatremia.

It is important to reiterate that getting enough water is still the main challenge for backcountry travelers. Exercising in extreme temperatures (hot or cold), dry climates, and high altitude all increase your fluid needs. If you are not acclimated to these environments you are more likely to lose excessive amounts of sodium in sweat. In warm, humid climates, be aware of how much you sweat, and consume a sodium-containing sports beverage or salty food periodically. One recommendation suggests one bottle of a sports beverage that contains electrolytes (not all sports drinks do) for every two bottles of water. The actual amount of total liquid will depend upon the length of time and intensity of the exercise.

In 2000, the American College of Sports Medicine (ACSM), the American Dietetic Association, and the Dietitians of Canada recommended the following: "Athletes should drink enough fluid to balance their fluid losses. Two hours before exercise 14 to 22 ounces of fluid should be consumed, and during exercise 6 to 12 ounces of fluid should be consumed every fifteen to twenty minutes depending on tolerance." Tolerance varies with individuals and, as was mentioned previously, this also differs with environmental conditions.

This water recommendation is not always practical in the backcountry, particularly if you are not using some kind of hydration pack. According to the curriculum director of the Wilderness Medical Institute of NOLS, Tod Schimelpfenig, aiming for 3 to 4 liters of water a day when backpacking in temperate climates is probably a good goal, assuming normal urine output. In conditions that increase your fluid needs, you can supplement plain water with warm drinks at camp, soups as part of meals, and by adding some drink mix to water periodically to increase your intake.

HYPONATREMIA PREVENTION STRATEGIES

- Know your body. Do you sweat excessively? Are you acclimated to the environment where you intend to travel or play?
- For exercise that lasts more than an hour (especially in the heat), plan to drink a combination of water and other beverages that contain both sodium and carbohydrates.
- If you take any medications or use other drugs, legal or otherwise, know if they increase your risk of hyponatremia.
- If you are small, slow, and sweaty during prolonged exercise, especially if you are not acclimated to an extreme environment, be aware.
- Know that there can be too much of a good thing.

CHAPTER 3

CARBOHYDRATES: YOUR BRAIN'S FAVORITE FOOD

If we could give every individual the right amount of nourishment and exercise, not too little and not too much, we would have found the safest way to health.

—Hippocrates, c. 460–377 B.C.

Eating enough calories (energy) and drinking enough fluid top the list of important nutrients for backcountry survival, but getting enough carbohydrates is part of making that jump from survival to enjoyment. While most athletes know carbohydrate foods are important for energy and performance, once outside of the athletic community, there is still a strong, though sometimes hidden, hesitation about carbohydrates. If you pay attention to only one thing nutritionally beyond calories and fluid in the backcountry, it should be carbohydrates.

Carbohydrates, commonly known as sugars and starches, are broken down into glucose (sugar) to fuel your brain and your muscles. The stored form of glucose is called glycogen. Muscle glycogen fuels physical activity, and liver glycogen fuels your brain and other cells as needed. You can store roughly 1,400 to 1,800 calories of glycogen in your body at a given time.

What is a Carbohydrate?

Carbohydrate: organic compound that contains various amounts of carbon, hydrogen, and oxygen molecules.

Simple Carbohydrate: (sugars) monosaccharides (glucose, fructose, galactose) and disaccharides (sucrose, lactose, maltose).

Complex Carbohydrate: (starch) three or more glucose molecules combined to form a polysaccharide.
Dietary Fiber: (carbohydrate polysaccharide) found in plant cell walls that humans cannot completely digest. Intestinal bacteria break down these compounds, and fiber keeps the digestive tract healthy.

This is enough stored carbohydrate to fuel roughly one to three hours of continuous moderate- to high-intensity exercise.

There are situations that will cause your body to use more glycogen in a shorter time span, such as carrying a heavy pack uphill, sprinting, high-altitude trekking or climbing, or exercising in a hot or cold environment. Fitness also plays a role since the more fit you are the more muscle you have and the more glycogen you can store (to a point). Sex is another factor that affects glycogen storage. Men typically have more muscle mass than women and can store more glycogen, so men need to eat more to fuel the extra muscle, but they may also be able to eat less frequently than their female expedition mates do.

In our bodies, the three sources of carbohydrate that provide energy for all body functions are blood glucose or blood sugar (5 grams or 20 calories), liver glycogen (75 to 100 grams or 300 to 400 calories), and muscle glycogen (300 to 400 grams or 1,200 to 1,600 calories). Roughly one hour of aerobic exercise uses over half of our liver glycogen supply, so with prolonged exercise, such as backpacking, climbing, or paddling in the backcountry, we depend upon our muscle glycogen stores for much of our energy needs. The depletion of muscle glycogen stores means muscle fibers lack the fuel needed to contract properly. This leads to muscle weakness, fatigue, and ultimately the inability to continue exercise, often referred to as "hitting the wall."

► Mix quick oats, peanut butter, your favorite dried fruit, and nuts and seeds for no-bake trail snacks. (For a real treat, add dark chocolate chips and put the treats someplace where the chocolate will melt; then let the chocolate harden again before eating—yum!)

When liver glycogen stores that feed the brain are depleted, the central nervous system reacts. This phenomenon is known as "bonking," the result of low blood sugar, and symptoms include irritability, dizziness, loss of focus, inability to concentrate, impaired vision, lack of balance, and disorientation.

► Chugging water at the end of the day to try to rehydrate is not a good idea. In addition to the fact that your body can absorb only so much at a time, this could fill you before you have eaten enough carbohydrates to replenish your glycogen stores. Sugar is fuel in the backcountry—you don't need to be afraid of it.

Carbohydrates are your brain's preferred fuel source, because they convert to blood glucose (blood sugar) faster than fat or protein. In fact, you need some carbohydrate to effectively burn fat for fuel. The saying in sports nutrition is that fat burns in a carbohydrate flame. No matter how much fat you may have stored, when you run out of stored carbohydrate (glycogen), you will experience fatigue and your performance will be affected. Also, if you deplete your liver glycogen and don't take in carbohydrate to keep your blood sugar steady, your performance will be negatively affected even if your muscles still contain glycogen.

The National Research Council has not established specific Recommended Daily Allowances (RDAs) for carbohydrate. Generally, sports nutrition experts recommend that athletes get 55 to 60 percent of total calories per day (400 to 450 grams per day) from carbohydrate sources. Some heavy endurance athletes consume diets with 70 percent of total calories from carbohydrates. A study of NOLS summer rations in 1999 at NOLS Rocky Mountain revealed that roughly 59 percent of the total calories were attributed to carbohydrates (see appendix E for more study details).

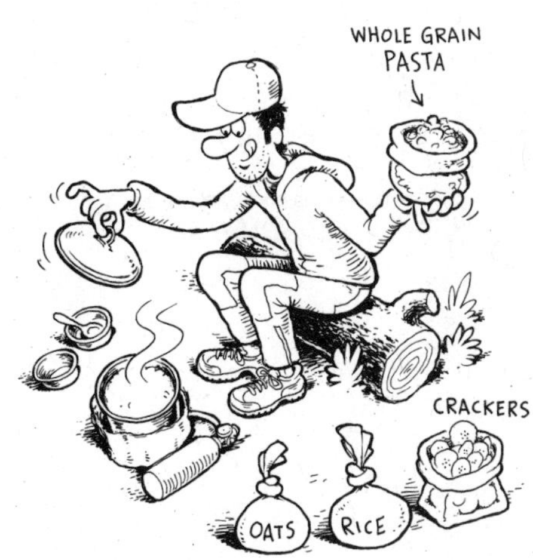

► If you have a sensitive digestive system and are worried about digesting beans in the backcountry, try taking Beano or another enzyme supplement to help your body adjust. Bean flakes and powdered hummus probably won't create a need for this enzyme, but it may help with mixes that contain textured soy protein (also called textured vegetable protein, or TVP).

Moderate exercise uses at least 50 percent carbohydrate for energy and high intensity exercise uses even more. As you increase your fitness, you will be able to use fat at a higher intensity level, but in the meantime, most moderate- to high-intensity efforts need more carbohydrates than fat for fuel. (And even when you increase your fitness, you need to maintain your blood sugar levels with carbohydrates during activity.) If you are breathing hard for whatever reason (lack of fitness, high altitude, or fast pace), your lungs cannot supply enough oxygen to match the exercise intensity and your body is forced to burn more carbohydrate than fat.

LOW BLOOD SUGAR

Low blood sugar or hypoglycemia occurs when the liver's supply of glycogen is spent and no carbohydrates are taken in to fuel the brain. Technically, hypoglycemia is a condition that occurs among persons with diabetes when blood sugar (glucose) drops to 40 to 50 milligrams per deciliter or lower (normal blood sugar is between 80 to 100 milligrams per deciliter). Basically, the brain needs glucose to function properly under normal circumstances. While your body can make glucose from parts of fats and proteins, this process is not fast or efficient compared to using carbo-

Symptoms of Hypoglycemia (Low Blood Sugar)

Dizziness
Confusion
Disorientation
Irritability
Weakness
Fatigue
Headaches
Extreme hunger
Anxiety
Fast heartbeat
Sweating
Shaking
Impaired vision

hydrates. Both stored glycogen and carbohydrate foods and drinks are quickly broken down for fuel. Symptoms of low blood sugar include dizziness, confusion, disorientation, irritability, weakness, fatigue, headaches, extreme hunger, anxiety, fast heartbeat, and, for some, sweating, shaking, and impaired vision.

> **► Leftover mini-pancakes (high in carbs) make great peanut butter sandwiches for trail snacks.**

In the backcountry, some of these low blood sugar symptoms can pose serious problems. Good judgment and a clear mind are crucial for the technical aspects of rock climbing, mountaineering, and navigating difficult hiking or boating terrain. Grumpy group members, suffering from low blood sugar, negatively affect group dynamics, creating unnecessary friction or adding to already tense situations. Watch for symptoms of low blood sugar in yourself and your group, especially if there are less fit or less experienced group members that may not realize how much fuel they need to function well in the backcountry.

> **did you know?**
>
> Low blood sugar increases cortisol levels. Cortisol is a hormone that can suppress immune function and contribute to an overtraining syndrome common among athletes.

Note for the Backcountry Professional

The degrees to which symptoms of hypoglycemia occur vary individually. Students or clients may not be accustomed to the level of physical challenge that a backcountry adventure provides, particularly the high intensity combined with longer duration, and low blood sugar symptoms may be a new experience. Educate students and clients about the symptoms early in the trip, and emphasize the importance of eating and drinking throughout the day to maintain blood sugar levels.

CARBOHYDRATE STRATEGY

There have been several studies conducted to determine the role of carbohydrate intake during endurance exercise. It is generally accepted from this research that people who exercise longer than ninety minutes benefit from carbohydrate intake during exercise. Food and beverages consumed during exercise may improve performance and help you feel better by maintaining more constant blood sugar levels. It is also important to replenish glycogen stores before and after exercise. Even if you take in carbohydrates while you exercise, there is no substitute for the high-carb meals at dinner and breakfast. Eating or drinking as you go will help with blood sugar levels, but glucose in the blood is not used as effectively as muscle glycogen for energy purposes.

> ▶ **Make your own "quick oats" by pulsing rolled oats in a blender or food processor (use this technique with rye, triticale, or barley flakes).**

Since backcountry adventures typically involve many hours of exercise on most days, it is important to keep up with the refilling of glycogen stores in order to keep blood sugar steady and muscles working efficiently. Many athletes are aware of the "magic window" for refueling; this refers to the fifteen-to-thirty-minute time period immediately following exercise when glycogen can be stored more easily. Combining some protein along with the carbohydrate helps repair injured muscle tissue along with filling the glycogen stores. For extended backcountry trips, taking advantage of this window of opportunity to refuel will help you feel better during multiple days of exercise.

> **did you know ?**
>
> Keeping your glycogen stores topped off on the trail (30 to 60 grams of carbohydrate per hour) can delay fatigue when exercise gets more intense and can help you tolerate cold climates better.

Often at the end of the day in the backcountry, getting to camp is either a time to rest after a grueling journey or time to set

Carbohydrates Prevent Fatigue

Low blood sugar, or hypoglycemia, and low glycogen stores are two causes of fatigue during exercise. Many studies of endurance sports show a benefit to blood sugar, performance, and the psychological perception of effort when carbohydrates are consumed during exercise lasting more than ninety minutes. Studies have also shown that pre-exercise carbohydrate intake may improve performance and delay the onset of fatigue when intensity levels are moderate to high.

How Much Carbohydrate Do You Need?

The recommendations for carbohydrates during exercise lasting more than ninety minutes is 30 to 60 grams per hour. A snack with water breaks is one way to do this in the field. Keeping an extra water bottle with drink mix that contains carbohydrates (sugar) is also helpful.

To replenish glycogen stores after moderate to heavy exercise, you need 8 to 10 grams of carbohydrate per kilogram of body weight. For example, if you weigh 60 kilograms ($60 \times 2.2 = 132$ pounds), you will need 480 to 600 grams of carbohydrate (1,920 to 2,400 calories) during the twenty-four hours following exercise. Combining food and beverages high in carbohydrates will help with this task.

Immediately following exercise, aim for at least $^{1}/_{2}$ gram of carbohydrate per pound (1 to 1.2 grams per kilogram) of body weight within the first thirty minutes. This will be somewhere between 50 and 100 grams (200 to 400 calories) for most backcountry travelers.

---

did you know ?

Training makes you able to use fat as fuel at higher intensity levels (this can spare some glycogen for later use). Well-trained muscle can store 20 to 50 percent more glycogen than untrained muscle.

up camp before dark. If rest is the first order of business, grab a snack that includes both carbohydrate and protein. Some good options include trail mix or a granola bar with nuts or seeds; peanut butter or cheese with crackers; or a water bottle with drink mix that is high in carbohydrate like a sports drink, lemonade, fruit punch, or any other mix available. If setting up camp is first on the list, eat a handful of nuts or seeds; then fill a water bottle with the drink mix to sip your carbohydrates as you get settled.

DIETARY FIBER

Found in plants, dietary fiber is a carbohydrate that humans do not possess the enzymes to completely digest. Soluble fiber in-

High Carbohydrate Backcountry Snacks

Food	***Serving Size***	***Grams of Carbohydrate***
Bagel	1	36
Hard candy	4 pieces	32
Drink mix	2 tablespoons	24
Fruit bar	1	28
Granola bar	1	24
Grape Nuts cereal	1/2 cup	38
Raisins	1/2 cup	57
Chocolate-covered raisins	1/2 cup	66
Yogurt pretzels	7 pieces	30
Fig bar	1 cookie	31

Copyright Beyond Broccoli Nutrition Counseling. Carbohydrate content may vary among different brands. Look at the labels of your favorite trail foods to find snacks with 30 to 60 grams for a realistic serving to meet your needs.

did you know ?

Eating more carbohydrates and less fat means eating more food to get enough calories for exercise (this may be a good thing to remind weight-conscious backcountry travelers who do not normally eat a vegetarian-type diet).

cludes gums and pectin found in oats, beans, peas, fruits, and vegetables. This type of fiber is metabolized by bacteria in the large intestine and can help lower blood cholesterol levels. Insoluble fiber such as cellulose, hemicellulose, and lignin, is not digestible. Insoluble fiber, found widely in whole grains, fruits, and vegetables, helps prevent constipation and other gastrointestinal problems.

The abundance of fiber available in many backcountry foods helps fill you up and contributes to keeping you regular in the field. Paying attention to what comes out of your body is a good way to monitor if you are getting enough fiber and fluid in the field. Soft, moist, easy to pass stool generally means you are hydrated

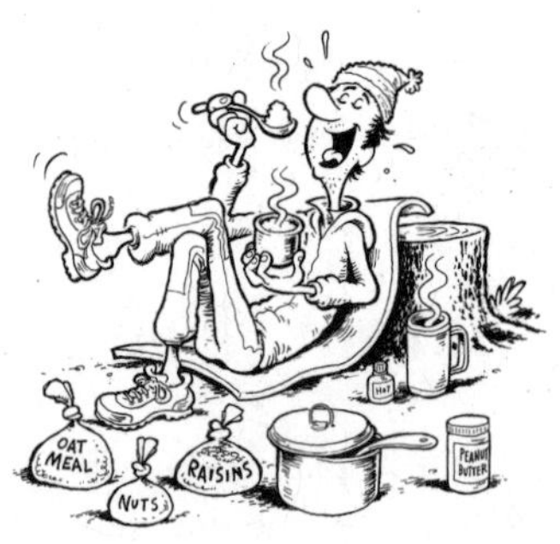

Alcohol is Not a Carbohydrate!

Contrary to popular belief, alcohol is not a carbohydrate. Alcohol in moderation may be a welcomed treat at the end of a hard day on the trail, but it is not a good energy source for replacing depleted muscle glycogen stores. Though alcoholic beverages are made from high carbohydrate foods such as potatoes, barley, and grapes, once these foods are transformed into an alcoholic beverage, they are no longer used as efficiently as other carbohydrates for fuel. Alcohol does yield 7 calories per gram (carbohydrates and protein yield 4, and fat yields 9 calories per gram), but the calories in alcohol contain no nutrients and can interfere with important metabolic processes such as replenishing glycogen stores.

well and eating plenty of fiber. Hard, dry stool is not only unpleasant to get rid of, but probably means you are dehydrated and may not be eating enough fiber. Remember that increasing fiber without enough fluid can cause constipation, bloating, stomach pain, and excessive gas. For some, eating too much cheese can also contribute to constipation. (See chapter 8 for more information about constipation and other digestive issues.)

OTHER FIBER FACTS

► Some good backcountry bread options (or bread substitutes) are bagels, pita pockets, corn tortillas, flat bread, and hard crackers.

Foods that are good sources of fiber also contain vitamins, minerals, and other components important for health.

Fiber slows the time it takes for food to leave the stomach (gastric emptying), thereby slowing glucose absorption in the small intestine. This helps control blood sugar levels and increases the feeling of fullness or satiety after a meal.

Fiber is related to a decrease in risk of certain cancers, coronary heart disease, obesity, diabetes mellitus, hypertension, and disorders of the gastrointestinal tract. (Good news for backcountry professionals who eat a high-fiber diet as their lifestyle!)

Dietary fiber recommendation: 20 to 35 grams per day (or 12 grams per 1,000 calories).

Adjusting to a High-Fiber Field Diet

Nutrition professionals advise clients to gradually increase the fiber in their diets to avoid possible gastrointestinal distress. In the backcountry you may not have this option.

Before going into the field, try to increase the fiber in your diet so your body will adjust more easily to a high-fiber field diet.

If you are having digestion issues (bloating, gas, cramping, or stomach aches), eat lower fiber foods and soups and drink lots of water to help your body adjust to a very high-fiber field diet.

Remember that dried fruits (in trail mix, fig bars, or by themselves) and veggies need extra water to digest properly.

Note: the average intake in the United States is 12 to 14 grams of fiber per day.

CARBOHYDRATE LOADING

did you know?

You use more carbohydrate for energy in high altitude and very hot or cold environments (burning fat requires more oxygen and more energy). Every gram of glycogen is stored with 2.7 grams of water.

Because many backcountry adventurers are also athletes, it seems wise to mention carbohydrate loading, a strategy sometimes used by athletes to prepare for endurance events. The traditional approach to "carb loading" begins the week before a long event. The athlete does a long workout to deplete muscle glycogen stores, followed by two to three days of a low carbohydrate diet to make sure the stores are as close to empty as possible. This depletion phase is followed by two to three days of a very high carbohydrate (and low fat) diet to fully replenish glycogen stores prior to the event. This practice has produced mixed results in scientific studies over the years and is currently not recommended by most sports nutritionists. Now the recommendation is to eat a diet high in carbohydrates and relatively low in fat for two to three days before a long event but to forget the depletion phase. If your backcountry adventure begins with a very long, strenuous day, then you may benefit from a few days of more carbohydrates than you normally would eat prior to the start of your trip. In general, however, making sure your backcountry diet is high in carbohydrates throughout the trip will be enough to help you feel and perform well, and carbohydrate loading will not be necessary.

Glycemic Index (GI)

Keeping blood sugar levels steady during exercise is important for athletic performance. In the backcountry, however, the focus goes beyond performance to include clear thinking, good judgment, positive mood, constant energy levels, and a strong immune system. The Glycemic Index (GI) is a system that ranks carbohydrate foods based on how they affect blood sugar levels. The GI was initially introduced to help people with diabetes figure out which foods would raise their blood sugar levels fastest. The system compares carbohydrate foods based upon the rate at which they increase blood glucose levels, using either 50 grams of glucose or white bread as the standard. High GI foods raise blood sugar levels fastest, and low GI foods raise levels more slowly. Many sports nutritionists use the GI system to guide athletes toward the best carbohydrate foods to consume before, during, and after exercise.

While this sounds reasonable at first glance, there are several problems with the Glycemic Index. The ability of food or drink to raise blood sugar (also called the glycemic response) is influenced by the amount of carbohydrate consumed, the fiber content, the amount of added fat, and the preparation of the food. We usually eat meals that contain a combination of carbohydrate, protein, and fat. Once a carbohydrate food is combined with protein and/or fat, the way that carbohydrate affects blood sugar also changes. For instance, baked potatoes are a high GI food, but once you add butter, sour cream, salsa, or just eat them along with a piece of chicken or meat, your blood sugar doesn't automatically rise the way it would if you ate just the baked potato by itself.

There are many other factors that affect the accuracy of GI ratings, including the amount of a food consumed (and more accurately, the amount of carbohydrate in the food). Carrots are the best example of this. Once again, carrots are a high GI food, but individual carrots are actually low in carbohydrate. So to create a high glycemic response, you would need to eat roughly a pound and a half of carrots—by themselves. Therefore a more useful (though still limited) application of the Glycemic Index takes the portion size and amount of carbohydrate into account to determine the Glycemic Load (GL). Unfortunately, while the GL system is more accurate, it is not a simple tool. You need to know the GI of the food and how much carbohydrate is in a serving of that food to calculate the GL.

Sports nutritionists that use the Glycemic Index (or Glycemic Load) advise athletes to eat moderate to low GI foods prior to exercise (with enough time to digest if the physical activity is high in intensity). High GI foods are better during and immediately after exercise when the body needs to break foods down quickly to keep the brain and muscles fueled. While this system can work pretty well for selecting grain foods that are high in carbohydrate and correspond more accurately with the GI rating than vegetables like carrots, it is still cumbersome to memorize lists of foods with various GI ratings.

An approach to proper fueling that may be more practical is to include foods with fiber, fat or protein, or some combination of these three components, prior to exercise for more sustained energy. Foods that contain fiber, fat, or protein are absorbed more slowly, and this helps control blood sugar, increases satiety after eating, and ultimately helps you stay satisfied longer after eating than low-fiber carbohydrates with no accompanying fat or protein (white bread, sugar candy, pancakes with syrup, or low fiber cereal). During and immediately after exercise are good times to eat these refined carbohydrates, because they break down quickly to fuel working muscles and brain, or to replenish depleted glycogen stores.

Depending on the day's activities, you may need easy-to-digest foods such as the refined carbs mentioned above, or it may not matter as much. During a high intensity day (uphill hiking or climbing, intense paddling through rapids, high altitude, or extreme heat or cold) you will benefit from carbohydrate foods that provide quick, efficient energy. For a more moderate pace or terrain, even if the day is long, carbohydrates are still key but getting some protein, fat, and fiber, along with your carbohydrates, shouldn't interfere with your performance and will provide more long-lasting fuel.

Glycemic Index of Some Common Foods

High (70 to 95)	***Moderate (55 to 70)***	***Low (15 to 55)***
Bagel, all types	Sucrose (table sugar)	Banana
Rice, instant	Raisins	Orange
White bread	Grape Nuts cereal	Bulgur
Honey	Oatmeal	Spaghetti
Instant potatoes	Orange juice	Milk, all types
Corn flakes	Soft drinks	Apple juice
Cheerios	Ice cream	Lentils
Carrots	Popcorn	Kidney beans
Hard candy	Wheat crackers	Chocolate
Rice cakes	Cornmeal	Peanuts

J. Benson and W. Askew. *Nutrition for Athletes*. Lifestyles Medicine, MA: Blackwell Science, 1999, 184.

CHAPTER 4 PROTEIN: MORE THAN MUSCLE

Life expectancy would increase by leaps and bounds if green vegetables smelled as good as bacon.
—Gary Larson, *The Far Side*

The latest rash of high protein, low carbohydrate diets has left many people with a fear of all things carbohydrate and an insecurity about meeting their protein needs. In fact, the original *NOLS Nutrition Field Guide* was written largely in response to a concern among NOLS students and staff regarding the amount of protein provided in the standard field rations. Since the standard NOLS rations are basically a lacto-ovo-vegetarian diet (a vegetarian diet that includes cheese, powdered milk, and eggs), it is a bit more difficult for those backcountry adventurers not familiar with this type of dietary regimen to identify which foods are providing protein.

Also in 2000, a nutrition survey that included both short-term and through Appalachian Trail (AT) hikers, many of whom did not necessarily follow a vegetarian diet, revealed a great deal of concern about getting enough protein (see appendix G for more about this survey). Even with opportunities to eat in towns along the way, AT hikers indicated that they craved protein foods, and one hiker commented, "I ate very little meat before the trip, and now I am a ravenous carnivore! I eat burgers and steaks in every town."

did you know?

Excess protein is either burned for energy or stored as fat.

Excess protein does not equal increased muscle mass. The only way to build muscle is to combine adequate protein with exercise that stresses your muscles.

► **Buckwheat groats (aka kasha) cook quickly and are a great substitute for ground meat in backcountry chili. Buckwheat is high in iron and a good source of B vitamins, potassium, magnesium, fiber, and the phytonutrient rutin that can lower blood pressure and cholesterol. Cook the groats first; then add water, tomato powder, Mexican spices, bean flakes, and dried onion to make chili.**

Many of the responses to this survey reflect common concerns and misperceptions about fueling extended backcountry travel. While there is no denying the importance of protein for endurance activities, it is relatively easy to get more than enough protein, even in the backcountry. For those who choose to eat a vegan vegetarian diet (no animal foods), some careful planning is necessary, not only for protein but for some important minerals best absorbed from animal sources (see chapter 11 for more about vegetarian diets). A backcountry vegetarian diet that includes some animal foods such as dairy, eggs, or fish, however, should have no trouble meeting both protein and mineral needs.

WHAT IS PROTEIN?

Proteins are a combination of amino acids that join to form various compounds that our bodies need to function properly. Our bodies can make all but nine of the amino acids needed in order to make these compounds. The nine amino acids it can't make, and therefore must get from food, are called essential amino acids. These essential amino acids are what concern vegetarians when they combine foods to form what is called "complete protein."

did you know 

Extra protein is needed during the early muscle-building phase of a backcountry trip (especially for those less fit), as well as during high intensity days in the field where tissue damage may occur, requiring protein to repair muscle.

There are a total of twenty separate amino acids; and, without exception, all natural, unprocessed animal and plant foods contain these twenty

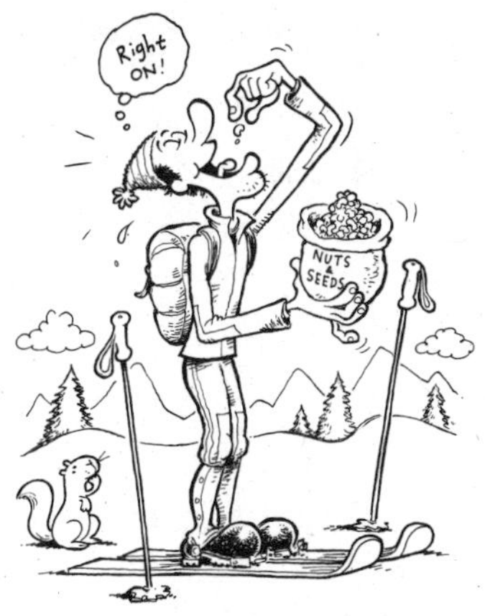

amino acids, but the amount of each amino acid in foods varies. Animal foods and soybeans are considered the most complete proteins since they contain adequate amounts of all amino acids needed to make new proteins. However, other plant foods such as grains, legumes, nuts, and seeds provide the necessary amino acids *only* when a combination of these foods is consumed throughout the day. Rice and beans or peanut butter on whole wheat bread are two common examples of food combinations that form a complete protein.

At one time we thought that the "incomplete" plant proteins had to be combined and consumed at each meal in order for our bodies to use the amino acids. We now know that these complementary protein foods do not have to be eaten at the same meal, as long as they are consumed within the same day. In other words, if you eat a variety of plant foods, including beans, nuts, seeds, and grains, you will get all of the amino acids that your body needs.

> ► **Add nuts and powdered milk to hot or cold cereal to make it last longer on the trail (this also adds protein, fiber, calcium, and good fats).**

FUNCTIONS OF PROTEIN

> **did you know ?**
>
> A variety of protein foods should be eaten throughout the day, especially if you are eating a strictly vegetarian diet.

There are very good reasons to be concerned about getting enough protein. The amino acids in protein foods are needed to make and repair muscle tissue, and they also produce the enzymes that facilitate various chemical reactions in the body, the hormones

Signs and Symptoms of Protein Deficiency	
Severe muscle wasting	Apathy
Weight loss or edema	Irritability
Dry, brittle hair that falls out easily	Anxiety
Skin lesions	
Dramatic loss of appetite (may or may not occur)	

did you know?

Since protein is more difficult to digest, meals and snacks eaten immediately before or during very intense exercise in the field should be high in carbohydrate, along with some protein (and little fat and fiber).

that are used to regulate many body processes, and the antibodies that protect us from disease and illness. Proteins also help maintain fluid and electrolyte balance, as well as acid-base balance; they play a role in blood clotting, and they transport fats, minerals, and oxygen within the body. Finally, proteins may be used as fuel if sufficient carbohydrates and fats are not immediately available.

Long strenuous days in the backcountry increase your need for protein. Part of this is due to a need for additional energy, especially if your glycogen stores are depleted and your brain needs fuel. Muscles can be broken down to provide the amino acid alanine that can then be converted to glucose for brain fuel. This is not an ideal situation, however, and it is part of the reason that eating and drinking a steady supply of carbohydrates during exercise is recommended to keep blood sugar steady—in order to fuel working muscles more efficiently.

► Red lentils cook fast (ten minutes or less) and are a great way to thicken soups while adding protein, iron, fiber, magnesium, potassium, and B vitamins.

Protein takes longer to digest than carbohydrate so when you include protein at meals and snacks, you will likely feel full longer than when you eat carbohydrate foods alone. This also means that if you are preparing for a strenuous day of intense exercise, you may want to eat only a small amount of protein and fat during meals and snacks to make sure that your body can properly digest the food. Because you cannot store protein, it is important to eat protein foods throughout the day to meet the high demands of backcountry exercise.

did you know ?

There is no evidence that more than 2 grams of protein per kilogram (.9 grams per pound) of body weight provides additional performance benefits.

RECOMMENDATIONS FOR PROTEIN INTAKE

The Recommended Daily Allowance (RDA) for protein for sedentary adults is roughly .4 grams per pound (8 grams of protein per kilogram) of body weight. Often you will see recommendations that use a percentage of total calories instead of a gram amount, and this is somewhere between 10 and 20 percent of total daily calories, depending on the source (high protein diet recommendations, for example, are typically 20 percent of total calories per day from protein). Many studies have examined the protein needs of athletes, and although there is still debate in this area, sports nutrition experts now recommend these amounts:

.5 to .75 grams of protein per pound (1.2 to 1.7 grams per kilogram) per day for recreational athletes

.6 to .9 grams of protein per pound (1.3 to 2 grams per kilogram) per day for competitive athletes, growing teenage athletes, and adults restricting calories or building muscle mass

While there are still questions about whether or not more than .9 grams per pound (2 grams per kilogram) provides any additional benefits, we do know that excess protein is not stored as protein. Just like excess carbohydrates and fat, any excess protein is stored as fat. There is no such thing as "protein (or amino acid) loading." This means you need to include protein every day, otherwise

► Try these creative protein snacks: tamari roasted almonds, curried cashews, cinnamon-covered walnuts, or cayenne pepper and honey roasted pecans.

Protein Recommendations*

Weight (lbs.)	*Weight (kg)*	*Protein/day (g)*
125	56.8	90
135	61	98
145	66	105
155	70	113
165	75	120
175	79.5	127
180	82	131
190	86	138

*Based on 1.6 g protein/kg/day

your muscles will be broken down to provide the amino acids your body needs for enzymes, antibodies, blood cells, and other important functions.

did you know?

Plant proteins may be combined at any time during the day—they do not need to be combined at each meal or snack to make complete proteins.

The increased need for protein among both endurance and strength athletes applies to most backcountry travelers who combine long days and strenuous activities. Higher protein needs are due to a combination of increased calorie needs for long and/or hard days of exercise, as well as the need to repair damaged muscle tissues or to build new muscle. Getting enough protein for the sedentary person or even the low end of a competitive athlete's requirements is not difficult with a varied diet, even in the backcountry. However, as protein needs increase, it is important to make sure protein is part of both meals and snacks throughout the day, particularly when the diet is plant based.

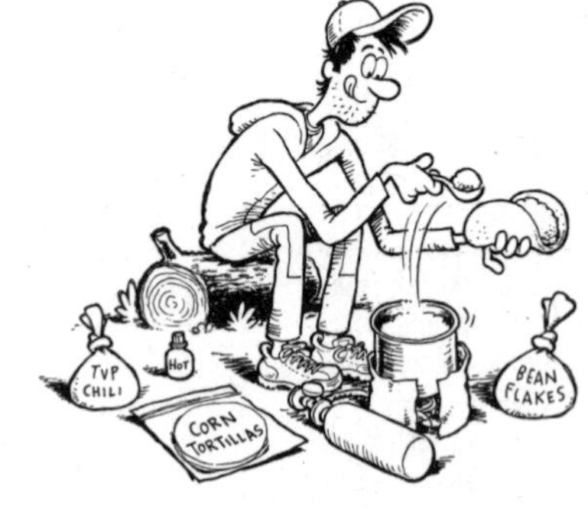

SOURCES OF PROTEIN

did you know?

Pasta, cereal, and other high carbohydrate backcountry foods provide a significant amount of protein.

When we think of protein, the main sources that come to mind are meat, poultry, fish, and eggs. Other sources include milk, cheese, nuts, seeds, beans, and legumes, as well as products made from legumes, such as tofu, veggie burgers, and hummus. A three-ounce piece of chicken or meat (roughly the size of a deck of cards) has about 25 grams of protein, while an egg, cup of milk, or ½ cup of cooked beans has roughly 7–9 grams. Grains are also a significant source of protein in the backcountry, and if combined with a variety of other foods (beans, legumes, nuts, seeds, dairy, or eggs), they provide all of the necessary amino acids to meet daily protein needs.

If your backcountry adventure includes fishing or you choose to bring jerky, canned meat, poultry, or fish, it will be even easier to meet your protein needs. This may be helpful at the beginning of an extended trip in the backcountry when you are building new muscle or during a winter trip where calorie needs are very high.

It isn't necessary to calculate your precise daily protein needs, not that you could without measuring your nitrogen balance anyway. However, it is a good idea to estimate a protein range for your size prior to going into the backcountry and then get some idea of how to meet those needs or at least know which foods are high in protein. If you are going on a NOLS course or other extended backcountry trip where rations are provided for you, familiarize yourself with foods that provide carbohydrates for energy and protein for keeping everything else in top form. You can also look at the sample field menus in appendix F to see what a day's worth of protein in the backcountry looks like.

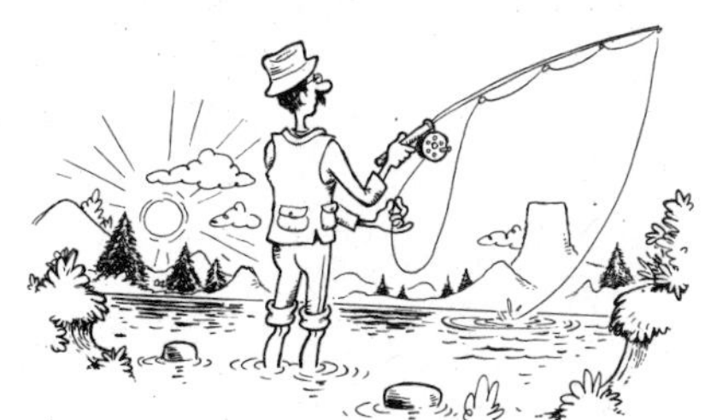

Backcountry Protein Sources

Food	***Serving Size***	***Grams of Protein***
Canned chicken	3 oz.	22
Canned sardines	1 can (4.25 oz.)	21
Chili mix	1/2 cup (dry)	20
Packaged/canned tuna	3 oz.	18 to 23 (varies with brand)
Packaged/canned salmon	3 oz.	18 to 20 (varies with brand)
Soy nuts	1/2 cup	18.5
Lentil soup mix	2/3 cup	17
Soy flour	1/2 cup	16
Falafel mix	1/2 cup (dry)	14
Tempeh	1/3 block	12
Cheese	1.5 oz.	11
Bulgur	1/2 cup	11
Buffalo jerky	1 oz.	10
Black bean mix	1/3 cup	10
Milk, from powder	8 oz.	10
Yogurt-covered peanuts	15 pieces	9
Veggie chili mix	1/4 cup	8
Peanut butter	2 Tbs.	7
Couscous	1/4 cup	7
Refried bean mix	1/4 cup (dry)	7
Egg, dried	1 Tbs. (= 1 egg)	6
Nutty Nuggets cereal	1/2 cup	6
Granola	1/2 cup	5 to 6
Quinoa	1/4 cup (dry)	5
Walnuts, raw halves	1/4 cup	5
Pasta and rice	1/2 cup (cooked)	3 to 4
Almonds, raw	12–15 nuts	2.8

High Protein Diets in the Backcountry

One evaluation during the 1999 NOLS rations study (see appendix E) included a full handwritten page regarding the amount of protein that should be considered for NOLS rations. The letter reflected the views of high protein diet proponents that have come in and out of vogue for the past forty years, most recently as the Zone Diet and Dr. Atkins New Diet Revolution. Both regimens advocate a dietary composition of 40 percent carbohydrate, 30 percent protein, and 30 percent fat compared to the general dietary guidelines that recommend 50 to 75 percent carbohydrate, 10 to 15 percent protein, and 30 percent or less from fat. Aside from the fact that this person had no idea how much protein was in the NOLS rations, this distribution of macro nutrients has not been favorably received by sports nutrition experts, given the plethora of research to support the benefits of higher carbohydrate intakes for endurance activities.

Currently sports nutrition research supports the idea that athletes need more protein than non-athletes do. As was mentioned above, the RDAs were not designed for the physically active minority in the United States. But claims that high protein diets are associated with increased athletic performance are not based on good science. High protein intake increases the need for water to get rid of the nitrogen byproducts of protein metabolism. We have already reviewed the challenge of staying properly hydrated in the field under normal circumstances (and learned that increasing fluid requirements to accommodate a high protein diet does not make sense).

Studies have also shown that after a few days of high protein and low carbohydrate intake, the acid buildup and decreased muscle glycogen impaired performance and caused fatigue. The carbohydrate section in this book addresses the importance of carbs for muscle glycogen stores, for performance, and ultimately for a sense of well-being that comes with steady blood sugar levels, as well as an adequately fueled brain and well-fueled muscles. It should also be noted that adequate overall energy intake, especially carbohydrates, improves nitrogen balance (an indicator of your protein status) and decreases protein requirements. If you don't get enough fuel, your body must break down muscle tissue in order to make glucose for energy. If you get enough calories and carbohydrates, your muscles stay intact.

CHAPTER 5 FAT: THE GOOD, THE BAD, AND THE UGLY

Hunger is the best sauce in the world.
—Cervantes, *Don Quixote*

Before high protein–low carbohydrate diets came back into favor, fat was the main dietary villain. While there are still many people who shun dietary fat in an attempt to achieve or maintain a healthy weight, carbohydrates have taken some of the spotlight from fat. We now realize that not all fats are equal with respect to health effects. The recommendations for fat intake have become more complicated as research related to essential fatty acids (omega-3s and omega-6s) and trans fats (partially hydrogenated oils) suggests the types of fat we take in may be as important as the amount. This poses some real challenges for backcountry travelers who want to extend their healthy everyday habits to their field diets.

If you are planning a single extended foray into the backcountry, you may be willing to make more nutritional tradeoffs related to the type of fats you eat than if you are a backcountry professional who spends many weeks or months of the year in the field. Chapters 12 and 13 discuss some of these considerations in more detail with respect to what happens when you come out of the field and also some special considerations for backcountry professionals. This chapter will give you some ideas about ways to balance realistic expectations of your backcountry fare and maintain good health.

FAT IS FUEL

Fat is a major source of energy (calories) for light to moderate exercise. Burning fat requires more oxygen than burning carbohydrate and, in fact, some carbohydrate is necessary to effectively burn fat for fuel. When you are kicking back at camp or traveling at a pace that allows comfortable conversation, you are most likely burning mainly fat. As the intensity of your exercise increases (setting a faster pace, climbing uphill, or carrying a heavier load) or you enter a higher altitude or extremely hot or cold environment, you will use more carbohydrate (glycogen) than fat. As your fitness increases, you will be able to use fat at higher intensity levels than when you are less fit, but glycogen is still going to be important because even when you are burning mainly fat, you always use a combination of fuels.

You can store much more fat than carbohydrate—100,000 calories worth or more—because fat cells are packed together without water. It is important to realize, however, that regardless of how much stored fat you have, if your liver stores of glycogen run out and your brain has to wait for fat or protein to be broken down for fuel, you are going to notice the effects. Your brain must have, on demand, the fuel it needs, and glycogen is its preferred source. Low blood sugar that results from depleted liver glycogen stores can make you feel crabby, hungry, tired, anxious, and confused (see the carbohydrate chapter for more details about low blood sugar). You can have plenty of body fat stored and even glycogen in your muscles, but if your brain is out of fuel, you will likely suffer.

THE MANY ROLES OF FAT

In addition to fueling body cells, fat has other important roles such as protecting your internal organs, insulating your body against temperature extremes, and transporting fat-soluble vitamins (A, D, E, and K). Fat is also important for transforming plant sources

> ► **For a trail mix rich in omega-3, include walnuts, soy nuts, or green pumpkin seeds.**

Functions of Fat

In the body

Provides energy (especially for low-intensity, prolonged-endurance activities)
Spares glycogen in fit individuals who can burn fat at a higher intensity
Forms body structures (cell membranes)
Helps make and/or transport fat-soluble vitamins (A, D, E, and K)
Insulates and protects organs
Helps regulate metabolic processes via hormones
Essential fatty acids protect the heart and brain; help decrease inflammation; and boost the immune system
Takes longer to leave stomach and is therefore more filling

In food

Provides more calories per gram than protein or carbohydrate (9 versus 4)
Provides taste and texture

of beta-carotene and related compounds into vitamin A as needed. Vitamin A is an important antioxidant, and in the backcountry, plant foods such as dried fruits and vegetables are major sources of this vitamin.

Fat in food provides calories for fuel and contributes to the flavor and texture of foods; and let's face it, taste is important. It takes longer for fat (and protein) to leave your stomach than carbohydrates. This makes meals and snacks that contain fat more satisfying and longer lasting than those with little or no fat.

The role that fat plays in backcountry nutrition varies somewhat according to the environmental conditions and the type of activity involved. Fat helps provide the large amount of fuel you need for winter or other high intensity expeditions, since fat yields 9 calories per gram compared to 4 calories per gram for protein and carbohydrates. A snack that includes fat can also help you stay warm at night in the field. On the other hand, excessive amounts of body fat make it more difficult for your

did you know?

Even a short-term increase in dietary fat that causes you to eat less carbohydrate can have a negative effect on your performance.

body to cool in hot environments. High altitude and extremely hot or cold environments can change how your body reacts to fat in foods; therefore, even though you may need fat to get enough calories, you may have to limit how much you can tolerate at one time.

► **Dehydrated salmon jerky, tuna, or wild salmon packets are great ways to boost your omega-3 intake in the backcountry (assuming you aren't able to fish). Add these to macaroni and cheese or pesto pasta for a meal.**

An excessive amount of fat may be harder to digest than carbohydrates, either prior to or during exercise. Too much fat during a day of heavy exercise (like loading up on cheese at lunch or on snack breaks) even at low altitudes and in temperate conditions can make you feel sluggish. The best approach is to include fat in both meals and snacks throughout the day but not to load up on it at any one time, especially if you need to continue exercising after eating. Eating an excessive amount of fat during a postexercise evening meal can also keep you from taking in enough carbohydrate to replenish your glycogen stores for the next day. This is one reason pasta with red sauce is a better postexercise meal than lasagna, especially if you must exercise the next day.

TYPES OF FAT

There are different types of fats and fatlike substances; together these compounds are called lipids. Triglycerides are the form of fat found in most foods and in the body. Sterols (such as cholesterol) and phospholipids are other fatlike compounds used to make and transport hormones and fat-soluble vitamins.

Types of Dietary Fats

Triglycerides (TG)—main fat found in food (fatty acid plus glycerol)

Cholesterol—not a fat but a lipid found only in animal foods; produced in our bodies, therefore not required in our diet.

Phospholipids—similar to triglyceride with a phosphate group added; not essential in diet, because we make them from TG.

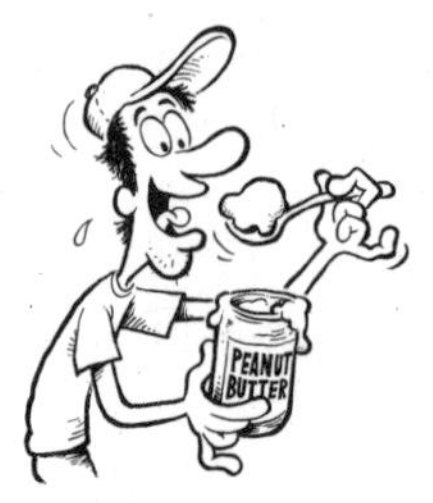

Though all of the various kinds of fat we eat and drink provide energy, the structure of the fat molecule affects how each type of fat impacts the body apart from providing calories. In general, trans fat made from partially hydrogenated oil should make up the smallest amount of dietary fat, followed by the saturated fats found in animal foods and tropical oils. The most beneficial fats for overall health are the unsaturated fats found in plant foods, fish, and seafood.

Many backcountry menus are mainly plant based and, therefore, supply mono- and polyunsaturated fats that provide health benefits, particularly for the heart. Nuts, seeds, various plant oils, grains, and legumes are all examples of foods with healthier fat profiles. Fruits and vegetables tend to have a minimal amount of fat, with the exception of avocados, which are high in the beneficial monounsaturated fat. Fish and certain nuts and seeds also contain beneficial fats called essential fatty acids, more commonly known as omega-3 fats.

Common backcountry sources of saturated fat include cheese, canned or dried meat, poultry, and fish. In NOLS rations, cheese is the main source of saturated fat (milk powder is nonfat, and egg powder is used mainly for baking). In addition to fat, however, these foods provide protein and important vitamins and minerals, satisfy you longer than meals without fat and protein, and help meals taste good, too. (Dietary fiber in carbohydrate foods also helps meals last longer.)

ESSENTIAL FATTY ACIDS

Essential fatty acids are special fats, including two that we must get from our diets. These fats provide key compounds for cell membranes, immune function, and vision, and are also related to both heart health and brain function. Essential fatty acids are particu-

> ► **Research shows that seeking comfort foods that are high in fat is a biological response to stress.**

larly important to the inflammation process, and chronic inflammation is now thought to play a major role in heart disease, diabetes, some cancers, Alzheimer's, and a host of other chronic diseases and conditions. Omega-3 (alpha-linolenic acid) and omega-6 (linoleic acid) fatty acids are the two fats we must get from food. Most plant oils are sources of omega-6s, and omega-3s are found in coldwater fish, flaxseed, walnuts, canola oil, soybeans, hempseeds (non-psychoactive variety), and purslane.

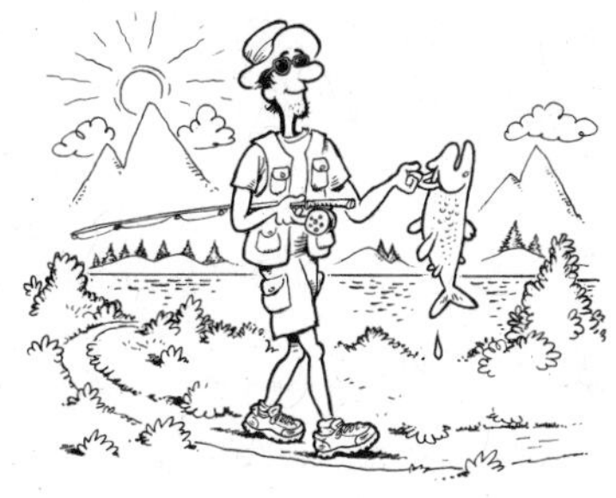

The impact these fats may have on backcountry travel is not known, but given the relationship between these compounds and the immune system, as well as functions of the brain and heart, it makes sense to incorporate foods rich in these fats when possible and practical. Unfortunately, the plant form of omega-3 is very susceptible to oxidation, so perishability is an issue. Flaxseeds, for example, need to be ground and kept in a sealed container, preferably away from direct light and heat. This care will allow ground flax to last three months in the refrigerator and indefinitely in the freezer, but the length of time in a backpack or other backcountry food storage container is not known.

TRANS FAT

An area of concern with respect to backcountry provisions, especially for outdoor professionals who rely on field rations for much of the year, is trans fat (aka partially hydrogenated oils). Trans fats are added to many processed foods to extend shelf life and contribute to taste and texture of certain foods. These fats are added to many cookies, crackers, and other snack foods, as well as more staple items such as peanut butter, bread, and packaged trail mixes.

did you know ?

Body fat and dietary fat are important in order to keep warm in cold climates.

did you know ?

It is more difficult to burn fat at high altitudes and when you are working hard, because of limited oxygen.

Trans fats are vegetable oils that have been processed to change the structure of the fat molecule. This allows the oil to become solid at room temperature (think margarine). At one time these oils were thought to be more nutritious than butter, but we now know these fats can increase the "bad" LDL cholesterol, decrease the "good" HDL cholesterol, increase triglycerides (another blood fat we do not want to be elevated), and contribute to chronic inflammation (another negative effect).

Although many manufacturers have omitted or reduced the trans fat in various products since the mandatory trans fat labeling went into effect in January 2006, these fats are still prevalent in many bulk food sources where a longer shelf life keeps food costs down for restaurants and institutional settings. Nutrition labeling is also deceptive in that a food that contains less than .5 grams of trans fat per serving can list "0 grams trans fat" and carry label claims such as "trans fat free" or "no trans fat." If the portion size of a food is in line with what you eat, then this labeling loophole probably isn't a big deal. The problem is that many snack foods list unrealistic serving sizes, and if the food is just slightly below the .5 gram cut off, the amount of trans fat you actually get (while thinking you are getting none if you have not read the ingredient list) can add up quickly.

RECOMMENDATIONS FOR FAT

General dietary recommendations for fat are usually given as a percentage of total calories. The dietary recommendations for Americans suggest a total fat intake of no more than 30 percent of total daily calories (that is, 600 calories or roughly 67 grams for a 2,000-calorie per day diet). Furthermore, less than 10 percent of total calories should come from saturated fat (looking at the 2,000-calorie per day regimen, that would be 200 calories from saturated fat or 22 grams).

Recommendations for Fat Intake

Lower limit for intake = 15% of total calories
Upper limit for intake = 30% of total calories
Saturated fat = 0% to 10% of total calories

World Health Organization. WHO and FAO Joint Consultation: fats and oils in human nutrition. *Nutrition Reviews* 53 (1995): 202–205.

The Dietary Reference Intakes (DRI) list acceptable total fat ranges as 20 to 35 percent for adults and 25 to 35 percent for children who are four to eighteen years of age. Recommendations revised in 2002 suggest roughly 10 percent of the total fat can come from the omega-3 and omega-6 fatty acids and that trans fat, saturated fat, and dietary cholesterol should be "as low as possible while consuming a nutritionally adequate diet." Many sports nutritionists recommend that athletes keep total fat to between 20 percent and 25 percent of total calories or .5 grams of fat per pound of body weight (1 gram per kilogram). A slightly higher fat intake in the backcountry (especially if it is the more desirable fats in foods like nuts, seeds, and grains) is appropriate, especially during trips that require a very high calorie intake.

ADAPTING TO A HIGHER FAT INTAKE

While your body is quite good at storing fat, adjusting to a higher fat diet is something some backcountry travelers wrestle with, particularly athletes accustomed to a low fat diet. If you find yourself in a backcountry cook group that likes to add a lot of fat to communal meals, you may experience gastrointestinal symptoms such as stomach aches, cramps, and constipation or just feel sluggish and more tired than usual after meals. This can also happen if you come out of the field

did you know?

Adding some fat to meals and snacks to make food taste good is important during cold weather and high-altitude expeditions, when appetite may be decreased and calorie needs are high.

> ► **Carry olive or canola oil in wide mouth containers when entering cold climates so you can get to it once it has congealed.**

and binge on fast food (or other high fat food) after extended time in the field.

Our bodies can adapt to more (or less) fat in our diet, but often this is not an immediate response. It can take several days for fat burning (aka fat oxidation) to match increased fat intake, according to the authors of at least one study that looked at the adaptation to a high fat diet.

Another important fact about fat as fuel is that trained athletes develop the ability to use fat as an energy source at higher intensity levels than untrained athletes. Several physiological changes that contribute to this adaptation involve enzyme activity, sensitivity to hormonal changes during exercise, increased use of ketones for fuel, enhanced fat transport throughout the body, and increased muscle triglyceride content. The bottom line is that, in trained athletes, these changes allow muscle cells to use free fatty acids more efficiently for energy production.

FAT PHOBIA IN THE FIELD

Given that we are living in a fat-phobic culture, it isn't surprising that a fear of eating fat shows up in the backcountry, often among women with concerns about body weight and shape. It is difficult to imagine how many extra calories you may need in the backcountry, depending on the many variables previously discussed, and even more difficult perhaps to visualize what that amount of calories looks like when applied to food. If you are used to watching your calories to either lose weight or maintain weight loss, you may be uncomfortable eating more fat than usual.

If you usually avoid high fat and high calorie foods, such as oil, butter or margarine, cheese, peanut butter, and granola, then it is unrealistic to expect that you will easily and automatically adjust to eating these foods when in the field. In addition to the biological adjustments your body may need to make so you don't experience the uncomfortable symptoms discussed above, your aversion to these high fat foods may be psychological and deeply ingrained. If you know prior to going into the field that you currently eat a low fat diet and that you have some issues with changing these patterns, it may be helpful to work through some of this ahead of time.

> **did you know ?**
>
> Your immune system benefits from omega-3 fats (cold water fish, flaxseeds, walnuts, canola oil, soybeans, and foods made from them).

It may help to learn why fat is so important in the field and to estimate how many calories and how much fat you will likely need, as well as what that amount of fat looks like in terms of food. Try to focus on fat as a fuel rather than something only associated with storage (excess body fat). If you are not in charge of choosing your rations or you are going to be part of a cook group in the field, you may need to make some adjustments. You may want to gradually increase your fat intake before you go into the field to help your body better adapt to your backcountry diet.

This justification of the additional calories may not be enough to resolve issues surrounding fat intake that go deep into the psyche, such as those related to eating disorders; however, often we hold on to ideas and habits without thinking about whether or not they are serving us well in the present

Why Is Fat Important in the Backcountry?

Fat can help you stay warmer at night or in cold environments.

Fat helps you meet higher energy (calorie) needs for both the obvious exercise (hiking, paddling, climbing, or skiing) and the more subtle life-maintenance tasks that require much more energy in the field (trekking between kiva or tent and bathroom or kitchen areas; hauling water for meal preparation; lifting heavy packs; or pulling sleds).

Fat is essential to keep your immune system strong, to produce hormones, and to get (and transport) important fat-soluble vitamins.

situation. In this case, understanding that eating fat does not immediately translate to unwanted weight gain and that not getting enough fat can negatively affect not only your backcountry experience but that of your expedition mates may be enough to spur a change in thinking—and habits.

There can also be some middle ground with respect to food preparation in the field. The group members at either extreme with respect to fat preferences may need to compromise. Obviously a 6′5″ male is going to need more calories than a 5′2″ female. Since fat is a good way to boost calories, the basic meal can be moderate in fat, and then high-fat ingredients like cheese can be added to individual portions rather than the whole pan. It is important to respect the food preferences and needs of your backcountry mates just as you respect their ideas and opinions.

SOURCES OF FAT IN BACKCOUNTRY FOODS

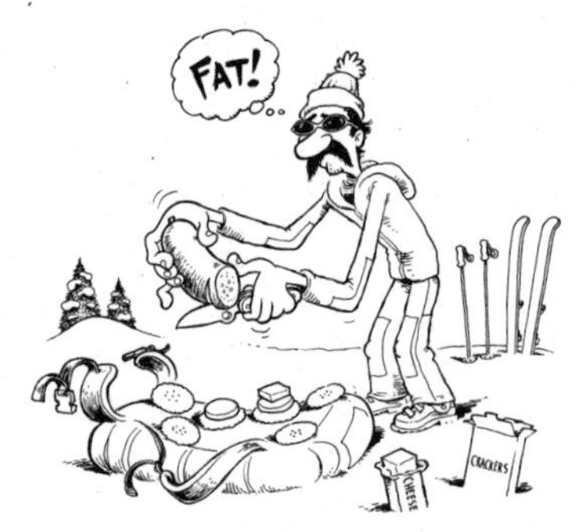

The discomfort you may experience during intense physical activity after excessive fat intake is one reason to be aware of snacks that should be eaten in moderation. There is a delay in the time when fat leaves the stomach (delayed gastric emptying) that may cause gastrointestinal distress (bloating, cramping, stomach pain). Cheese and peanut butter are obviously high in fat, but sources such as malted milk balls may be less obvious. These are foods that may not digest well during heavy exercise, so it may be best to eat less of them or to combine them with lower fat foods for meals and snacks.

The sources of fat in backcountry rations are pretty straightforward, as you can see in the table. The majority of fats in these foods are the unsaturated varieties that are recommended in place of saturated fat.

Sources of Fat in Backcountry Foods

Food Item	*Serving Size*	*Amount of Fat (grams)*	*Type of Fat**
Honey-roasted peanuts	1/4 cup	18	M/P/S
Peanut butter	2 Tbs.	16	P/M/S
Vegetable oil	1 Tbs.	14	P/M/S
Malted milk balls	5 pieces	12	S/T
Margarine	1 Tbs.	11	P/M/S
Sesame sticks	1 oz.	11	P/M/S
Cheese, cheddar	1 oz. (1″ cube)	10	Mostly S
Granola bar	1	10	P/M/S
Cheese, jack	1 oz.	9	Mostly S
Sunflower seeds	2 Tbs.	9	P/M/S
Yogurt pretzels	7 pieces	8	S
Granola	1/2 cup	7	P/M/S
Roasted soy nuts	1/4 cup	6	P/M/S
Cracker mix	1 oz.	6	P/M/S

*Types of fat: **M** = monounsaturated, **P** = polyunsaturated, **S** = saturated, **T** = trans fat

FAT IN NOLS RATIONS

As mentioned above, NOLS backcountry rations consist largely of plant-based foods rich in the healthier types of fats. Prior to the publication of the first *NOLS Nutrition Field Guide,* many students and instructors perceived cheese to be a mainstay of NOLS rations and were concerned about the amount of fat this staple provided. According to a survey conducted in the NOLS Rocky Mountain rations department during the summer of 1999 (see appendix E for more about this study), the total fat content of the rations was roughly 31 percent of total calories, and the saturated fat content was less than 10 percent. Both of these levels were (and remain) in line with nutrition recommendations.

Of course, since the NOLS rations are bulk provisions, some students eat more of various foods than others, and it is

did you know ?

Endurance training increases the size and number of mitochondria (and oxidative enzymes) in cells, which allows athletes to use more fat during workouts at a higher intensity.

possible to overeat cheese (particularly if you have a cook-group mate that eats less cheese, making more available for the rest of the group). However, cheese provides some protein and calcium and is a versatile, tasty (if you like it) addition to meals and snacks. This is yet another example of how eating in the field may diverge from everyday eating patterns out of the field. While there are many foods that provide protein, calcium, and a more beneficial fat profile than cheese does, adding cheese to a backcountry meal can increase the enjoyment of it, and the importance of enjoying food also must be a consideration. Cheese is a familiar food, and during a time when you are adjusting to a new environment and a different diet, perhaps even learning how to cook for the first time, familiar foods may be helpful psychologically.

CHAPTER 6

VITAMINS, MINERALS, AND PHYTONUTRIENTS: THE SMALL STUFF THAT MATTERS

Difficult as it may be to believe, eating more vitamins or minerals than are needed does not make healthy people healthier.
—Marion Nestle, *What to Eat*

The final segment of nutrition basics includes vitamins and minerals (also called micronutrients), as well as the emerging category of important plant compounds called phytonutrients. Vitamins and minerals do not provide direct energy or form cell structures like the macronutrients (carbohydrate, protein, and fat), but they are involved in nearly every reaction in the body. As cofactors, these compounds help your body absorb, process, and use the energy from carbohydrates, protein, and fat; support your immune system; deliver oxygen and nutrients to cells; and strengthen muscles and bones, just to name a few.

Phytonutrients are compounds that protect plants and often give fruits and vegetables their bright colors or strong flavors. These compounds tend to be more involved with various processes that prevent disease such as lowering blood cholesterol levels; controlling chronic inflammation, blood sugar, and blood pressure; fighting cancer cells; and protecting vital organs such as the heart, brain, and eyes. The role phytonutrients play in backcountry nutrition is related to the many antioxidant compounds that assist the body during periods of physical and psychological stress, helping to keep things in balance. The good news is that many foods commonly taken into the backcountry are full of phytonutrients, including legumes, dried fruit, coffee, tea, and chocolate.

GETTING ENOUGH VITAMINS AND MINERALS

Many health conscious people preparing for an extended trip ask about the need to take supplemental vitamins and minerals into the backcountry. There are some variables to consider such as the length of time you will be in the backcountry, the foods you choose to pack, and any preexisting conditions that may predispose you to a deficiency of something (history of anemia or the need for a medication that depletes nutrients). If you follow a strict vegan diet or other restrictive food regimen, you may also want to make sure your backcountry provisions provide all of the essential nutrients (see chapter 11 for more information about special diets).

In general, if you are healthy prior to your trip and you eat and drink enough calories through a varied diet to sustain your backcountry activities, it is unlikely you will develop a vitamin or mineral deficiency in less than a month (or more). Extreme environments may increase your need for some nutrients, such as sodium and potassium (which are electrolytes that are lost in sweat) or the antioxidants that help your body keep excessive free radicals produced from exercise, high altitude, and sun exposure in check. Even these situations do not automatically mean you need to lug bottles of pills along, but they do reinforce the idea that carefully planning your backcountry menu is wise.

Reasons for Low Vitamin or Mineral Intake

Not enough calories to fuel activity
Restrictive diets due to:
- food allergy
- food intolerance
- food preferences (vegan diet, low carbohydrate, low fat, picky eater)

Excessive mineral losses due to sweat or illness
Higher needs due to shivering, illness, etc.
Poor planning—not enough variety to balance nutrients
Reliance on highly processed foods that are low in nutrients

► **If venturing somewhere during berry season, research the edible varieties that you may find so you can enjoy this incredible source of vitamin C, fiber, and many different phytonutrients.**

Food is generally thought to be the best source of most nutrients due to beneficial synergistic effects. Synergy refers to the way many different compounds in food work together to nourish or protect us. Isolated individual nutrients studied in pill form often don't produce the expected results. One explanation for this is synergy. The bottom line is, contrary to what the supplement industry would like you to believe, no one really knows enough yet to ditch food in favor of supplements. Plus, supplements are more likely than food to provide too much of some vitamins and minerals that have negative health effects when taken in excess (one food exception is liver, which can provide excessive amounts of vitamin A). There are situations when supplements may be helpful, and these will be addressed later in this chapter. But, in general, you are much better off keeping your focus on food sources, especially since getting enough calories and water are still the most important nutritional goals in the backcountry.

The need to plan menus that include easy-to-pack foods that cook fast and use a minimal amount of fuel and water leads to some nutritional tradeoffs. Refined carbohydrate foods that have been enriched or fortified (meaning either some of the nutrients lost in processing were added back or more nutrients were added than the original grain) are an example of such a tradeoff. This can actually be beneficial in some cases since fortified foods may add folate, iron, calcium, and vitamin B_{12}; these are nutrients that may be hard to get enough of in your backcountry diet. But relying solely on processed foods is not a good idea since the enrichment and fortification processes don't add all of the original nutrients (such as vitamin E, the mineral selenium, and some of the B vitamins) and tend to contain less dietary fiber than their whole-food counterparts. One approach is to balance refined carbohydrate foods with dried fruit and vegetables, nuts and seeds (and butters made from them), bean flakes (and other products made from legumes), and some of the whole grains that cook

► **For a change of pace and an excellent assortment of vitamins, minerals, and phytonutrients, try adding dried dates, plums, figs, or apricots to trail mix and hot or cold cereals.**

quickly such as bulgur, oatmeal, rye flakes, buckwheat groats, quinoa, and whole-wheat couscous.

The end of this chapter includes tables for various vitamins and minerals including what each compound does, how much you need (including the upper intake levels so you don't get too much), what happens if you don't get enough, and food sources. The recommended amounts of nutrients in this chapter use the RDA (Recommended Daily Allowance) as well as the Tolerable Upper Intake Levels (UL). The RDAs were established to prevent nutrient deficiencies; however, they may be low with respect to optimal levels of some nutrients, but they do provide a basic guideline. The popularity of various dietary supplements and fortified foods has increased the likelihood that we may get too much of some nutrients; therefore, this table includes the UL for nutrients that may be a problem in excess. Since none of these recommendations are specifically designed for very (or extremely) active people, the rest of this chapter will discuss some of the nutrients you may need beyond the RDA amounts.

EFFECTS OF FOOD PROCESSING ON NUTRIENTS

Backcountry rations depend largely upon dehydrated fruits, vegetables, beans, and other processed foods to provide nutrition in a form conducive to multi-day expeditions (lightweight, easy to pack and prepare, and long-lasting). Questions surrounding the nutritional value of these processed foods arise often. While various nutrients in food are affected by exposure to oxygen, light, extreme temperatures, and acidity, there are actually some foods that are enhanced by processing. Beans and legumes are two examples of food where heat breaks down compounds, such as fiber and protein, allowing them to be digested more easily. Other nutrients may be absorbed and used more easily by the body when heated, such as certain B vitamins and carotenoids (a family of plant compounds, some of which we convert to vitamin A as needed).

► **Vegetarian cookbooks and magazines are a great resource to teach you how to use a variety of herbs and spices.**

The nutrient most affected by processing is vitamin C (ascorbic acid). Much of the vitamin C may be lost (10 to 50 percent) due to light, copper, iron, or dissolved oxygen. Losses of water-soluble B vitamins during drying average 5 percent. Some items, such as the tomato powder and drink mixes used in the NOLS rations, are good sources of vitamin C. There are other commercial drink mixes, such as Tang, that contain vitamin C.

Minerals are less affected (or not affected at all) by freeze-drying or dehydrating. In fact, dehydrated fruit is often a concentrated source of the minerals iron and potassium. Many common dried or dehydrated backcountry foods are also good or excellent sources of phytonutrients (see the table on page 72 for foods high in phytonutrients).

The key is to balance processed foods that may lack some nutrients with a variety of grains, nuts, seeds, dried fruits, and vegetables. Enjoy fresh foods when they are available: forage wild edibles using a trusted guide; fish, hunt, arrange for fresh fruit or veggies for a meal at reration sites; or seek fresh foods in towns when resupplying provisions. But know that many of the foods that must be processed in order to survive your backcountry journey are still nutritious choices. The emphasis placed on the value of fresh whole foods versus the highly processed foods that have become staples of the American diet is valid. However, keep in mind that there is a difference between the highly processed fare found in fast food restaurants and the dried fruits, veggies, legume-based meal mixes, and refined grains used in the field. Backcountry nutrition must be viewed differently, taking into account the high level of physical activity involved and the fact that even without predominantly fresh food on the menu, there are many highly nutritious foods, some whole and some that have been processed for convenience and the reality of backcountry living.

ANTIOXIDANTS

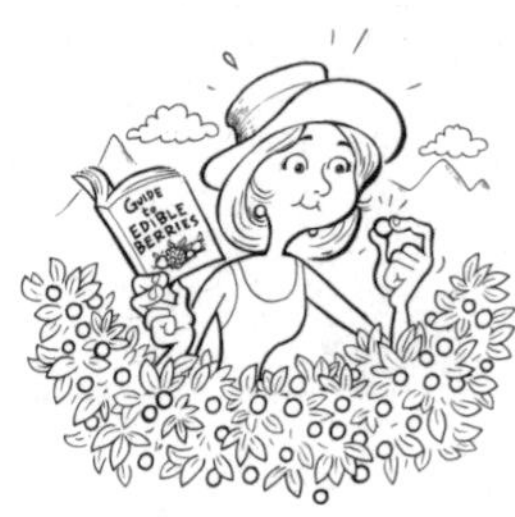

The term antioxidant is widely used, often to sell supplements or to coax people into eating more fruits and vegetables, yet most have no idea what antioxidants are or why we need them. If you pay attention to the marketing materials for various antioxidant supplements, you may think we have things sorted out in terms of how much we need, which forms are best, and what they do for us; and you may think that you need pills in order to get enough of them. Research dedicated to antioxidants over the past decade or so paints a different picture, with mixed results as to whether or not these nutrients protect us against heart disease, cancer, and other chronic diseases. Even the role antioxidants play in exercise performance and muscle recovery is murky.

Backcountry adventures include many situations that cause our bodies to produce cell-damaging compounds, such as excessive and strenuous physical activity, exposure to sun, high altitude, and a variety of physical and psychological stresses. Antioxidants are one of the ways our bodies deal with these potentially damaging compounds. But some of these seemingly problematic compounds are also part of our immune system, with the power to protect cells, and they may even repair muscle tissue. Confused? You are not alone. This section will give you an overview of what antioxidants are and why they are of interest to backcountry travelers.

Antioxidant Terms

Free radical: highly reactive molecule with an unpaired electron in its outer shell (superoxide and hydroxyl radicals); part of immune system but can also cause cell damage.

Reactive Oxygen Species (ROS): substances related to but not officially free radicals; compounds that contain oxygen and have the ability to damage tissues (hydrogen peroxide and singlet oxygen).

Antioxidant enzymes: produced by body to neutralize free radicals (superoxide dismutase (SOD), glutathione peroxidase (GPX), and catalase).

WHY WE NEED ANTIOXIDANTS

The high level of exercise in the backcountry means your body is using a lot of oxygen (or you are at high elevations with not enough oxygen, also a problem). A natural part of breathing oxygen leads to the formation of unstable, highly reactive compounds. Some of these compounds are called Reactive Oxygen Species (ROS) and others are called free radicals. Our bodies usually keep these potentially dangerous compounds in check by making special antioxidant enzymes and using various antioxidant vitamins (A, C, E), minerals (selenium), and phytonutrients (special compounds in plant foods) from the foods we eat or supplements we take. Oxidative stress is the term used to describe the situation where too many of these reactive compounds are formed for your body to deal with them appropriately. Left unchecked, these compounds can damage cells and may be related to fatigue, tissue inflammation, muscle soreness, and delayed healing from injuries.

Radicals Generated by Muscular Contraction
Superoxide
Hydrogen peroxide
Nitric oxide
Hydroxyl radicals

In addition to breathing more oxygen, other factors that contribute to oxidative stress include exposure to chemicals found in food and water, radiation (including UV sun exposure), pollution, drugs, ozone, hypoxia (lack of oxygen), tobacco smoke, and other stresses. Currently, oxidative stress has been linked to a variety of chronic diseases such as heart disease, Alzheimer's, cataracts, and certain cancers. The links of interest to backcountry travel include postexercise muscle damage, fatigue, immune system function, and problems adapting to high altitude.

The good news for highly active backcountry adventurers is that trained athletes appear to make more of the antioxidant enzymes that are used to keep reactive molecules in check. So making sure you get the minerals selenium, copper, and zinc that your body uses to make these enzymes can help you keep things in balance, especially in the beginning of your trip when your body is adapting to higher levels of exercise. In addition to the antioxidant enzymes, eating a variety of antioxidant-rich foods may also help your body deal with or prevent oxidative stress.

Backcountry Foods High in Antioxidant Nutrients (Including Phytonutrients)

Berries (fresh and dried)
Buckwheat groats (kasha)
Cereals
Coffee
Cocoa (chocolate)
Dates
Dried cranberries
Dried plums (prunes)
Figs
Flaxseeds
Garlic
Herbs and spices (many if not all)
Legumes (black and kidney beans, lentils, etc.)
Milk (powdered and fortified with vitamins A and D)
Olive oil
Onions
Peanuts
Seeds (sesame, pumpkin, poppy, sunflower, etc.)
Soy (soy nuts, TVP, etc.)
Tea (green, black, oolong)
Whole grains (oats, quinoa, buckwheat)

ANTIOXIDANT SUPPLEMENTS

Studies have tested various antioxidant supplements to see if they can prevent oxidative stress, as well as some of the negative effects of this condition, like muscle soreness, but the results have been mixed. Some research shows antioxidant supplements, such as vitamin E, can enhance the body's response to oxidative stress; others show no significant differences. Even the studies that show a decrease in indicators of stress don't show improvements in exercise performance.

Reactive Oxygen Species

ROS (Reactive Oxygen Species) are compounds produced during strenuous exercise that may damage cells and play a role in muscle soreness. Like free radicals, however, ROS also play important roles in the body. ROS are related to muscle contractions and other adaptations to training, and may even help heal muscles. In addition to keeping free radicals in check, antioxidant foods, phytonutrients, supplements, and enzymes may help maintain a balance of ROS.

A recent study looked at vitamin C supplements as a way to decrease postexercise muscle damage and to delay muscle soreness. The results showed less of the reactive oxygen species (ROS) thought to cause the muscle damage in the vitamin C group, but no difference in muscle soreness. Furthermore, vitamin C slowed the recovery of muscle function, suggesting that these ROS may actually play a role in muscle recovery. In fact, the much-maligned free radicals that we try to eliminate with antioxidants are another important part of the immune system, with the capability to destroy viruses and bacteria. Free radicals are also involved in radiation and chemotherapy used to fight cancer cells, as well as the production of prostaglandins that play a role in cell growth and pain regulation. This is where things get really murky.

There are many theories to explain the mixed results in antioxidant studies but no definitive answers. Vitamin E is actually a family of compounds, and yet many studies use the one compound thought to be the most biologically active—alpha-tocopherol. Going back to the earlier discussion about synergy, which is the way various compounds in food work together, it is possible that even though the other members of the vitamin E family aren't as active, they are still important. There is also

> ▶ **Energy bars are often part candy bar, part multivitamin. If you like them, they can provide easy, quick snacks on the trail. If you don't like them, leave them home and eat real food that you enjoy.**

the possibility that inflammation, not oxidation, is the real culprit in muscle damage, so the antioxidants did not address the problem of reducing inflammation. Another reason may be that a variety of antioxidants are needed, rather than just one or two high-dose supplements. Whatever the reason, it is important for you to know that there are still more questions than answers with respect to antioxidant supplementation and oxidative stress.

Backcountry travel usually involves both strenuous and prolonged physical activity, and we know such efforts produce potentially damaging compounds. We don't know for sure that our body's antioxidant system is enough to keep pace with this type of effort, but we do know that some of these reactive compounds may have beneficial effects. Since good backcountry nutrition aims to help both performance and overall health, it seems wise to include a variety of foods that provide antioxidant nutrients. There is an added bonus with the food-first approach, in that many of the foods rich in antioxidants also have anti-inflammatory, antiviral, antibacterial, and anticancer effects, or they can lower cholesterol or blood pressure (see the Phytonutrients: Special Plant Compounds table at the end of this chapter). Many of these plant foods are also good sources of a variety of vitamins, minerals, and dietary fiber, all of which play an important role in backcountry health and well-being.

If you are planning an extended expedition in an extreme environment, such as high altitude, a multivitamin and mineral supplement is a reasonable addition to your backcountry supplies. This would provide a range of antioxidants, as well as iron, zinc, vitamin D, and the B vitamins we don't store in appreciable amounts, to support any dietary shortcomings or increased needs. There is some research to support the theory that higher doses of vitamin E than you can easily get from food (see the vitamin E section of this chapter) may be beneficial, but the results are still not completely clear.

VITAMINS—A BRIEF OVERVIEW

The two basic types of vitamins are water soluble and fat soluble. The water-soluble vitamins include vitamin C and the family of B vitamins—thiamin (B_1), riboflavin (B_2), niacin (B_3), pyridoxine (B_6), cobalamin (B_{12}), pantothenic acid, and folate. These vitamins are absorbed in water and with the exception of B_{12} are not stored in large amounts in the body. The fat-soluble vitamins include A, D, E and K. Fat-soluble vitamins require fat to be properly absorbed (this is one reason you need to take your multivitamin supplement with food) and in the case of vitamins A and D may be highly toxic in large doses.

WATER-SOLUBLE VITAMINS

The fact that water-soluble vitamins are not stored as extensively as the fat-soluble vitamins, and some of the excess is excreted in urine, has led to the myth that there are no dangers associated with getting too much of the water-soluble vitamins. In fact, excess B_6 can cause a loss of feeling in the fingers, excess B_3 can cause a burning and flushing sensation, and excessive vitamin C can cause diarrhea (not a pleasant backcountry experience).

B Vitamins

The B vitamins are crucial for energy production, and the higher amount of energy required to live and travel in the backcountry means your needs for these vitamins may be higher than they are out of the field. Luckily, many backcountry foods such as whole and enriched or fortified processed grains (breads, cereals, pasta, etc.), nuts, seeds, and legumes are all good sources of many of the B vitamins. Vitamin B_{12} is an exception since all of the natural sources are animal foods. The common backcountry foods naturally rich in B_{12} include cheese; jerky; canned meat, poultry, or fish; and powdered milk. Plant sources of B_{12} do not contain a form that humans can use. but there are many vegetarian foods that are fortified with B_{12} (see chapter 11 for more information about vegetarian diets and nutritional yeast that contain B_{12}).

Vitamin C

Vitamin C is an important antioxidant vitamin that also plays a role in forming connective tissue called collagen and helps your body absorb the iron found in plant foods. Vitamin C is abundant in fresh fruits, including many wild berries and vegetables, but it is easily destroyed by heat and exposure to air. This means dried fruits and veggies are likely to have little, if any, vitamin C. Powdered tomato and fortified drink mixes, such as the ones issued by NOLS, are an easy way to add this important vitamin to your backcountry rations.

The amount of vitamin C needed for optimal health remains controversial. While the upper limit for vitamin C is 2,000 milligrams per day (200 milligrams per day is thought to be enough to saturate body tissues) there are researchers that believe these amounts are not accurate because during situations when your body needs more vitamin C, higher levels are tolerated. Studies of high dose vitamin C supplementation and endurance performance have yielded inconsistent results. While some studies showed improvements in strength, there were also decreases in endurance. Studies have looked at a possible link between vitamin C and post-exercise muscle soreness, but again the results are mixed (see antioxidant section). Some studies have shown that vitamin C can reduce the severity and duration of colds, but it does not prevent them altogether.

Since excessive amounts of vitamin C can cause diarrhea (as mentioned previously, not a good situation in the backcountry) and in some people increase the risk of developing kidney stones, the backcountry doesn't seem like a good place to experiment with high-dose supplementation. If in the past you have used powdered vitamin C packets to flavor water, during or following physical activity, with no ill effects and you like the taste of these packets, they may be a good way to get some vitamin C and increase your fluid intake in the field.

FAT-SOLUBLE VITAMINS

As mentioned in the introduction to vitamins, fat-soluble vitamins need fat in order to be properly absorbed. This is one reason it is recommended that you take your multivitamin supplement following a meal (assuming most meals contain a mixture of fat and other nutrients). Vitamins A and D are also among the nutrients that may be harmful in high amounts.

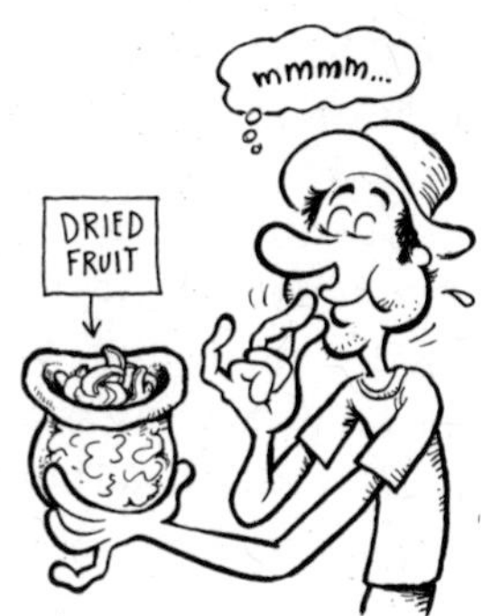

Vitamin A

Vitamin A is a powerful antioxidant that comes in a variety of forms. The active form of vitamin A found in animal foods and many supplements is called retinol. Liver, egg yolk, cheese, whole or fortified milk, and fish oil are sources of retinol. Beta-carotene (as well as some other carotenoids, there are more than 600 of them) can be transformed to vitamin A in our bodies as needed. Carotenoids are found in orange, red, and dark green plant foods such as fruits and vegetables. Even dried fruits such as apricots are good sources of beta-carotene (the drying process destroys some, but apricots have so much to start with that they remain a great source).

Eating excessive amounts of vitamin A from animal or fish liver (or the liver oils) has proved fatal on at least one expedition (though there is some controversy surrounding this), but it is more likely that you could get too much of this vitamin from supplements. Unless you are hunting animals to eat, in the backcountry you are most likely to get your vitamin A from plant sources such as dried apricots and mangoes or fortified foods like powdered milk, margarine, or butter.

Vitamin D

Vitamin D helps us absorb calcium and is best known for its role in bone health. More recently this fat-soluble vitamin has been linked to muscle strength, cell growth, chronic inflammation, and immune system function. Current research has discovered vitamin D receptors in nearly every cell of the body, suggesting a much larger role than was previously thought. Vitamin D is not a major concern for the majority of backcountry travelers that spend many hours in the sun, since most people are able to synthesize vitamin D with just ten to fifteen minutes of unprotected sun. The caveats are that many people now diligently and wisely use sunscreen, older adults produce less vitamin D from sun exposure, and people with darker skin need more sun exposure to make D. Also, people that live and travel in northern latitudes may not be able to make enough vitamin D during the fall and winter months, even with otherwise adequate sun exposure.

Since vitamin D is a fat-soluble vitamin that our bodies store, it was assumed that getting enough sun—throughout the spring and summer months—provides enough to get us through the winter. Recent studies show low vitamin D levels in northern climates: some areas include Seattle, Washington, and Boston, Massachusetts, in the U.S., as well as many places in Canada. Low levels have been found even among people who use sunscreen in temperate climes or who have limited access to the outdoors. If you are planning an extended winter trip it may be worth getting your vitamin D levels tested (blood levels of 25-OH D or calcidiol).

Fatty fish, egg yolk, liver, and fortified foods such as milk and some cereals are food sources of vitamin D. The new information about vitamin D has led to more fortification of foods since few foods are naturally high in this vitamin.

In 2007 a group of international researchers published a call for regulatory agencies to increase the recommendations for vitamin D. The current RDA is 200 to 400 international units (IU) (5 to 10 micrograms per day) for adults under seventy years of age. The tolerable upper limit for vitamin D is currently 2,000 IU (50 micrograms per day). Meanwhile, many vitamin D experts recommend 1,000 to 1,500 IU per day (25 to 35 micrograms per day) from a combination of foods and supplements. Some experts include a safe, limited amount of sun exposure in addition to foods, but many are opposed to recommending sun exposure due to the known risk of skin cancer associated with unprotected sun exposure.

Vitamin E

Vitamin E is one antioxidant that has shown the ability to affect both oxidative stress and chronic inflammation related to exercise and has been particularly interesting in high-altitude situations. One of the arguments in favor of vitamin C supplementation is that it helps recycle vitamin E. Vitamin E, or more accurately the vitamin E family that includes four tocopherol and four tocotrienol compounds, is one possible exception to the need for antioxidant supplements.

It is difficult to get more than the Recommended Daily Allowance (RDA) for vitamin E from food sources alone. The RDA for vitamin E is 15 milligrams per day, but the current suggestions for antioxidant benefits of vitamin E are around 200 to 400 milligrams per day. Food sources of vitamin E are mainly plant oils (found in nuts, seeds, and whole grains). One tablespoon of plant oil contains 3 to 5 milligrams of vitamin E and 135 calories (15 grams of fat). So if you want to get roughly 400 milligrams from plant oil, you would consume 10,000 calories and 1,200 grams of fat. Even if the benefits of vitamin E were clearer for these high dosages, natural food sources are not the answer, given this amount of fat and calories.

On the positive side, natural food sources contain the whole vitamin E family rather than the alpha-tocopherol found in most supplements. Researchers suspect that some of the mixed results in vitamin E studies may be related to the fact that we need the whole vitamin E family to get the same benefits seen in studies where people get vitamin E from foods.

If you venture into the backcountry for an extended period of time at high altitude, it may be worth taking a vitamin E supplement or a multivitamin supplement that includes vitamin E. High-altitude travel can decrease appetite, and very high altitude may make fat digestion more difficult. Since vitamin E occurs naturally in high fat foods, this could pose a challenge at high altitude. There is some interesting research regarding vitamin E supplementation well above the RDA (400 milligrams per day). Vitamin E may decrease lipid peroxidation, one of the processes that damages cells at high altitude and may be detrimental to health and athletic performance.

MINERALS—A BRIEF OVERVIEW

There are many minerals important to backcountry nutrition, some of which are highlighted below. Nuts, seeds, beans, legumes, dried fruits and vegetables, cheese, powdered milk, canned or dried meat, poultry, and fish or other seafood are all good sources of minerals. Processing, such as dehydrating or canning, does not deplete minerals, and many processed foods commonly taken into the backcountry are especially high in sodium. This is an example of a nutrient that is needed often in much higher amounts in the backcountry than in everyday life out of the field. (The water and extreme environment chapters discuss sodium in more detail.)

In general, mineral deficiencies are not likely to develop in the field if enough calories from a variety of foods are consumed, assuming you begin your journey in good health. Vegetarians, particularly vegans that eat no animal foods, may need to carefully examine their rations to make sure they include foods rich in zinc, calcium, and iron since these minerals may not be as prevalent or easy to absorb in common backcountry foods. (See chapter 11 for more information about special diets.)

IRON

Iron is an important mineral for the production of red blood cells and the myoglobin that delivers oxygen to working muscles. Iron deficiency can cause endurance problems for athletes and is also linked to poor immune function, fatigue, short attention span, irritability, and poor learning ability.

Iron in food occurs in two forms: heme and nonheme. Heme iron is found only in animal foods and is available to the body in greater amounts than its nonheme counterpart. We absorb 10 to 35 percent of the heme iron from foods and only 2 to 10 percent of the nonheme iron. Nonheme iron is found in both animal and plant sources but is the only iron in plant foods. Vitamin C increases the absorption of nonheme iron by preventing the oxidation of ferrous iron to create ferric iron (ferrous iron is better absorbed). Adding tomato powder to bean and legume dishes or drinking vitamin C-fortified drink mixes with meals will help you absorb more iron from your backcountry meals that tend to rely on nonheme iron.

If you have a history of iron-deficiency anemia, it is a good idea to have your iron levels checked prior to venturing into the backcountry for an extended trip. Low iron can make you feel fatigued, especially if your trip involves high-altitude travel, and if your iron stores are low, you may want to take a supplement along. If you are a woman with a history of iron-related anemia, perhaps due to excessive monthly blood losses from menstruation, a multivitamin and mineral supplement may be appropriate especially if you are spending more than a month in the field. You may not need to take the supplement daily, but it may be helpful during your period. Some women experience changes in menstrual flow in the field, either losing significantly more blood or having no period at all.

Although iron is important for red blood cell formation, and the needs for red blood cells increase with both endurance activity and high-altitude exercise, the evidence regarding iron deficiency without anemia does not consistently show impaired performance. If you do not have a known iron deficiency, however, iron supplements are not a good idea. Excessive amounts of iron are stored in the body and can cause damage to cells.

High Iron Backcountry Foods

Serving Size/Source	***Mg of Iron (% RDA)****
1/2 cup Nutty Nuggets cereal	14.4 (80%)
3 Tbs. cream of wheat (dry)	9 (50%)
1 cup raisin bran cereal	4.5 (25%)
1/3 cup black beans	2.7 (15%)
1/4 cup falafel	2.7 (15%)
3/4 cup bowtie pasta	2.7 (15%)

*RDA 18 mg; % based on 2,000 calories per day

Minerals at a Glance

Iron is needed to form hemoglobin in blood and myoglobin in muscle that deliver oxygen to cells throughout the body.

Magnesium is involved in more than 300 enzyme reactions and is important for bone health, muscle contractions, making various proteins, using glucose, and many other vital roles.

Calcium and at least eight other minerals (plus a couple of key vitamins) contribute to bone strength and many of these minerals, including calcium, are also important for muscle movement and coordination. Calcium is also essential for transmitting nerve impulses and blood clotting.

Sodium, chloride, potassium, magnesium, and calcium function as electrolytes, keeping body fluids and acid-base balance in check.

Selenium, zinc, and copper are an important part of antioxidant enzymes used to balance free radical and other compounds that can damage cells during exercise. Zinc plays a major role in wound healing and other immune system tasks as well as being part of many enzymes used to produce energy.

PHYTONUTRIENTS

In addition to vitamins and minerals, there is another class of nutrients that we are just beginning to understand called phytonutrients. Phytonutrients are special compounds found in plant foods and appear to be protective for both plants and humans. While there is no research at this point to support a specific backcountry advantage of phytonutrients, the role these compounds play, related to boosting the immune system and exerting both antioxidant and anti-inflammatory effects, suggest they are beneficial.

See the tables on pages 72 and 83 for lists of many of the foods that contain phytonutrients, and the table on page 83 for information about some of the roles these compounds play with respect to human health. In addition to fruits, vegetables, grains, beans, legumes, nuts, and seeds, some other sources of phytonutrients are many herbs and spices, which not only help to flavor food but also help you to avoid boredom (also known as "flavor fatigue"). These phytonutrients are another reason a spice kit can be an important part of your backcountry kitchen on an extended trip.

Backcountry Spice Kit

Dry	Liquid	Other flavoring options
Salt and pepper	Soy sauce	Pesto mix
Cinnamon	Vinegar	Taco seasoning packets
Curry powder	Olive oil	Parmesan cheese
Italian seasonings	Hot sauce	Sesame seeds (or gomasio)
Mexican seasonings		Dried seaweed
Cayenne pepper or red chili flakes		Nutritional yeast
Dried onion flakes		
Garlic powder		

Phytonutrients: Special Plant Compounds

Phytonutrient	*What it does*	*Food Sources*
Thiols:		
Allyl sulfides (allicin, isothiocyanate, sulforaphane)	• Suppress cholesterol production • Lower blood pressure • Deactivate some hormones that promote tumor growth • Trigger detoxification enzymes in the liver	Onion and garlic families (onions, leeks, scallions, shallots, garlic, chives), broccoli, cauliflower, watercress, cabbage, kale
Phenols:		
Flavonoids (Anthocyanins and anthocyanadins)	• Prevent binding of carcinogens to DNA • Anti-cancer properties	Red and purple fruits and vegetables (berries, eggplant, plums, red cabbage), red wine
Catechins, phenolic acids (ECG, ECGC)	• Neutralize free radicals	Green, black, and oolong teas; dark chocolate, red wine, berries

Phytonutrients: Special Plant Compounds (continued)

Phytonutrient	*What it does*	*Food Sources*
Flavanols (quercetin, rutin, myrietin, kaempferol)	• Neutralize free radicals • Anticancer properties	Apples, tea, onions, buckwheat, berries, apricots, dark chocolate, dates, dried plums, figs, citrus
Stilbenes (reservatrol)	• Lower cholesterol • Anticancer properties • Antiviral properties • Anti-inflammatory actions	Grapes, peanuts, red wine, blueberries, cranberries
Phytoestrogens Isoflavones (Genistein, diadzen)	• Mimics estrogen action • Lowers total cholesterol and raises HDL • Anticancer effects	Soybeans and soy products (small amounts in other legumes, grains, and vegetables)
Lignans	• Anticancer properties • Weak estrogen-like effects • May have antoxidant effects	Flaxseed, asparagus, broccoli, carrots, whole grains, some berries, many nuts, seeds and legumes
Curcuminoids (curcumin)	• Anti-inflammatory • Antioxidant activity • May have anticancer effects	Turmeric (curry powders, yellow mustard)
Plant Sterols:		
Sterols (beta-sitosterol, campesterol, stigmasterol)	• Cholesterol-lowering effect • May reduce tumor growth	Soy, peanuts, rice bran, berries, beans and legumes, nuts, seeds, whole grains

Terpenes:		
Carotenoids (lutein, beta-carotene, zeaxanthin, lycopene—over 600 different compounds!)	• Antioxidant • Cancer-fighting • Some may protect the macula • Help repair DNA	In most yellow, orange, red, and green fruits in vegetables—beets, cantaloupe, apricots, mango, spinach, kale, sweet potatoes, tomatoes
Limonenes	• May deactivate certain carcinogens • Activates detoxification enzymes	Peel of citrus fruits
Geraniol	• Antioxidant • May have anticancer effects	Bergamot, coriander, nutmeg, carrots, lavender, blueberry, blackberry, lemon, lime
Glycosides:		
Saponins	• May lower cholesterol • Anticancer properties • Antioxidants	Alfalfa, beans, chickpeas, lentils, soy, whole grains, potatoes, onions, garlic, leeks
Other compounds:		
Capsaicin	• Anticoagulant (blood clotting) • May protect DNA • May kill *H. pylori* (bacteria that causes stomach ulcers) • Clears nasal congestion	Hot chili peppers, cayenne pepper
Indoles (indole-3-carbinol)	• Converts active estrogen to inactive form • Protective against some cancers	Cruciferous vegetables—broccoli, cabbage, kale, brussels sprouts, watercress, cauliflower

WHAT TO DO IN THE FIELD

The decision to take supplements in addition to food into the backcountry for extended trips to ensure an adequate intake of nutrients remains somewhat controversial. Getting enough calories through a variety of foods that contain the various nutrients important for backcountry travel is probably enough for most people. If you are traveling into extreme environments (especially high-altitude and cold climates) or have dietary restrictions that limit your food choices, a multivitamin and mineral supplement is not a bad idea. Many people have lost sight of the fact that supplements are just that, supplemental, and not intended to replace food. If you plan an overall fairly nutritious menu and are able to eat and drink throughout the day, taking a supplement a few times a week may be enough to make up for the nutrients that you may need in slightly higher amounts than you are getting from food. There are also many foods that are fortified with vitamins and minerals, such as cereals, that may be better than supplements because they also provide calories, macronutrients (carbohydrates, protein, and some fat), and dietary fiber.

Vitamins

Name	*RDA*[1] *UL*[2]	*Major Functions in Body*	*Major Sources*	*Deficiency Symptoms*
Fat-soluble vitamins				
Vitamin A (retinol, β-carotene)	M 900 μg F 700 μg M and F 2,800 to 3,000 RE (retinol equivalent)	Skin and mucous membrane tissue, night vision, bone development, immune function	Retinol: animal foods (fish, egg yolk, cheese, whole or fortified milk and other dairy foods) Carotenoids: orange and yellow vegetables and fruits; dark green leafy vegetables; fortified margarine	Night blindness, intestinal infections, impaired growth
Vitamin D[3]	5 to 10 μg (200-400 IU) 50 μg[3] (2,000 IU)	Bone and tooth formation, calcium absorption, muscle strength, cell growth, immune function, thyroid and insulin function, possibly anti-inflammation	Fatty fish, egg yolk, liver, fortified dairy and other foods; also produced in skin from UVB light	Rickets (children), Osteomalacia (adults) —both rare in U.S. (low blood vitamin D levels seen in autoimmune disease and many cancers)
Vitamin E	15 mg 800 to 1,000 mg	Antioxidant to protect cell membranes	Plant oils (corn, nut, seed, soy, olive, etc.), sunflower seeds, nuts,legumes, green leafy vegetables, whole-grains, wheat germ, egg yolks, margarine	Very rare: disruption of red blood cell membranes, anemia

Vitamins (continued)

Name	RDA[1] UL[2]	Major Functions in Body	Major Sources	Deficiency Symptoms
Fat-soluble vitamins				
Vitamin K	M 75 to 120 μg F 75 to 90 μg ND	Blood clotting	Eggs, liver, green leafy vegetables; intestinal bacteria	Increased bleeding, hemorrhage
Water-soluble vitamins				
Vitamin C	M 75 to 90 mg F 65 to 75 mg 1,800–2,000 mg	Collagen formation (connective tissue), iron absorption, formation of epinephrine, antioxidant	Citrus fruits, green leafy vegetables, peppers, potatoes, dried tomato powder, fortified drink mixes, energy bars and cereals	Weakness, rough skin, slow wound healing, bleeding gums, scurvy
Thiamin (B_1)	M 1.2 mg F 1.0 to 1.1 mg ND	Energy production from protein, fat, carbs; central nervous system and heart function	Whole-grains, rice bran, enriched grains (bread, pasta, cereals), meat, pork, legumes, wheat germ	Poor appetite, apathy, mental depression, fatigue, pain in calf muscles, edema, beriberi

Riboflavin (B_2)	M 1.3 mg F 1.0 to 1.1 mg ND	Energy production from carbs and protein; healthy skin maintenance	Milk, cheese, fish, poultry, eggs, enriched grains, green leafy vegetables, beans, and meat	Dermatitis, cracks at corners of mouth, sores on tongue, damage to cornea
Niacin	M 16 mg F 14 mg 30 to 35 mg	Energy production from carbs—anaerobic and aerobic conditions; fat metabolism; healthy skin	Whole and enriched grains, beans, fish, poultry, red meat, nutritional yeast, cheese, dates, peanuts, potatoes, broccoli, carrots, corn; also made in body from tryptophan (an essential amino acid)	Loss of appetite, weakness, skin lesions, canker sores, fatigue, indigestion, gastrointestinal problems, pellagra
Vitamin B_6	M 1.3 to 1.7 mg F 1.2 to 1.3 mg 80 to 100 mg	Protein metabolism; formation of hemoglobin and red blood cells; breakdown of glycogen; production of glucose from protein and fat	Protein foods: legumes, fish, poultry, meat; whole grains; green leafy vegetables; nutritional yeast; peanuts; sunflower seeds; walnuts; oats; carrots; avocados	Nervous irritability, convulsions, dermatitis, sores on tongue, anemia, seizures
Folate	400 μg 800 to 1,000 μg	DNA formation; red blood cell development	Green leafy vegetables, whole and fortified grains, broccoli, nutritional yeast, dates, cheese, chicken, lentils, mushrooms, oranges, fruits, legumes, nuts	Fatigue, mental confusion, gastrointestinal problems, diarrhea, anemia; neural tube defects in newborns

Vitamins (continued)

Name	RDA* / UL	Major Functions in Body	Major Sources	Deficiency Symptoms
Water Soluble Vitamins				
Vitamin B_{12} (cobalamin, cyanocobal-amin)	2.4 μg / ND	Formation of DNA; red blood cell development; nerve tis-sue	Animal foods: fish, clams, cheese, milk, eggs, meat, poultry; nutritional yeast, and some fortified foods	Pernicious anemia, nerve damage

[1]**Recommended Daily Allowance (RDA)**—amount of nutrient needed daily for most healthy people to avoid developing a deficiency. Ranges given include 14 to 18 yrs (low end of range) and 19 to 50 yrs.

[2]**Tolerable Upper Intake Levels (UL)**—the maximum level of daily nutrient that is likely to pose no risk of adverse effects. Includes intake from food, water, and supplements. Due to lack of data, ULs are not determined (ND) for vitamin K, riboflavin, vitamin B_{12}, pantothenic acid, biotin, or carotenoids.

[3]**Current** recommendations for vitamin D are based on adequate intake levels (AI) and do not include sun exposure. These values are also controversial; a group of international researchers published a request in 2007 to increase the requirements for vitamin D. Many experts now believe adults need a minimum of 1,000 IU/day and that 2,000 IU/day should not be the UL.

Major and Trace Minerals

Name	*RDA** *UL*	*Major Functions in Body*	*Major Sources*	*Deficiency Symptoms*
Major Minerals				
Calcium (Ca)	1,300 to 1,000 mg 2,500 mg	Bone formation, enzyme activation, nerve impulse transmission, muscle contraction, cell membrane potential	Milk, cheese, egg yolk, canned fish with bones, dried beans, figs, oats, almonds, sesame seeds, tofu, dark green leafy vegetables	Osteoporosis, rickets, impaired muscle contraction, muscle cramps
Phosphorus (P)	1,250 to 700 mg 4,000 mg	Bone formation, acid-base balance, cell membrane structure, B vitamin activation, component of organic compounds (ATP, etc.)	All protein foods—meat, poultry, fish, eggs, nuts, seeds, milk, cheese, dried beans; whole grains and dried fruits	Rarely occurs: similar to Ca deficiency, muscular weakness, brittle bones
Magnesium (Mg)	M 410 to 420 mg F 360 to 320 mg 350 mg (UL applies to supplement form only)	Protein synthesis, metalloenzyme, glucose metabolism, smooth muscle contraction, bone component	Fish, milk, dried beans, nuts, whole-grains, many fruits and vegetables, nutritional yeast, tofu, sesame seeds	Rarely occurs: muscle weakness; apathy, muscle twitching, muscle cramps, cardiac arrhythmias

Major and Trace Minerals (continued)

Name	*RDA** / *UL*	*Major Functions in Body*	*Major Sources*	*Deficiency Symptoms*
Major Minerals				
The following major minerals have adequate intakes (AI) not RDAs:				
Potassium (K)	4,700 mg ND	Positive ion in intracellular fluid; glucose transport into cell; same functions as sodium but intracellular	Found in most foods; abundant in bananas, dried fruit, vegetables, potatoes, milk, fish, and meat	Hypokalemia, loss of appetite, muscle cramps, apathy, irregular heartbeat
Sodium (Na)	1,500 mg 2,300 mg	Positive ion in extracellular fluid; nerve impulse conduction; muscle conduction; acid-base balance; blood homeostasis	Small amounts in most natural foods; significant amount in canned, dried and packaged foods (1 teaspoon salt contains 2,000 mg sodium)	Hyponatremia, muscle cramps, nausea, vomiting, loss of appetite, dizziness, seizures, shock, and coma
Chloride (Cl)	2,300 mg 3,600 mg	Negative ion in extracellular fluid; nerve impulse conduction; hydrochloric acid formation in stomach (protein digestion, B_{12} metabolism)	Widely distributed in foods; intake associated with sodium (table salt combines Na and Cl)	Rarely occurs: convulsions; may be caused by excess vomiting and loss of hydrochloric acid (HCl)

Trace Minerals				
Iodine (I)	150 µg ND	Formation of thyroid hormones	Iodized salt, seafood, fish, milk; iodine water purification tablets	Goiter, enlarged thyroid gland
Iron (Fe)	M 11 to 8 mg F 15 to 18 mg 45 mg	Hemoglobin and myoglobin formation, electron transfer, oxidative processes	Fish, meat, poultry, eggs, nutritional yeast, dried plums, dried beans and peas, whole and fortified grains, pumpkin and sesame seeds, dates, raisins, green leafy vegetables. *Also available from iron cookware.*	Fatigue, anemia, impaired temperature regulation, decreased resistance to infection
Selenium (Se)	55 µg ND	Cofactor of glutathione peroxidase (antioxidant)	Brazil nuts and whole grains, vegetables and nuts grown in Se-rich soil; fish, meat, shellfish, onions, wheat germ	Rare: cardiac muscle damage
Zinc (Zn)	M 11 mg F 9 to 8 mg ND	Energy production, protein synthesis, immune function, sexual maturation, taste and smell sensations	Milk, cheese, nuts, eggs, whole grains, vegetables, legumes, fish, meat, poultry, mushrooms, pumpkin, sunflower seeds	Depressed immune function, impaired wound healing, depressed appetite, failure to grow, skin inflammation

Major and Trace Minerals (continued)

Name	*RDA** *UL*	*Major Functions in Body*	*Major Sources*	*Deficiency Symptoms*
Trace Minerals				
Chromium (Cr)	M 35 μg F 24 to 25 μg ND	Enhances insulin function (glucose tolerance factor)	Cheese, corn, eggs, mushrooms, dried beans, potatoes, whole grains, organ meats, nutritional yeast, beer and wine	Glucose intolerance, impaired lipid (fat) metabolism
Copper (Cu)	890 to 900 μg ND	Use of iron and hemoglobin in body, connective tissue formation and oxidation reactions	Nuts, shellfish, eggs, seeds, cheese, cocoa powder, oats, lentils, whole grains, salmon, fish, broccoli, raisins, green leafy vegetables	Osteoporosis, inability of body to make collagen, fatigue, baldness, slow growth
Fluoride (F)	M 3.0 to 4.0 mg F 3.0 mg ND	Formation of bones and teeth	Drinking water, canned salmon, tea, seafood	Higher incidence of dental cavities
Manganese (Mn)	M 2.2 to 2.3 mg F 1.6 to 1.8 mg ND	Enzymes involved in energy metabolism; bone formation; fat synthesis	Whole grains, dried beans and peas, nuts, seeds, nutritional yeast, figs, tea, wheat germ, cocoa, apricots, dairy	Poor growth

Molybdenum (Mo)	43 to 45 μg ND	Works with riboflavin in enzymes involved in carbohydrate and fat metabolism	Whole-grain products, dried beans and peas, organ meats	Not found in humans
Boron (B)	Essentiality likely, but not proven yet; estimated requirement 1 to 13 mg	Steroid hormone and vitamin D, hydroxylation reactions	Fruit, vegetables, nuts, cinnamon, beans, and whole grains	Decreased estrogen and testosterone, increased Ca and Mg losses, bone loss, impaired mental and immune functions

*RDA values based upon 2004 National Academy of Sciences recommendations for males and females ages 15 to 50 years of age. If one value is given, it is the same recommendation for both genders. If a range is given, it is in the order in which it appears from 15 to 50 (10 to 5 μg = 10 μg for females 15 years of age and 5 μg for females 50 years of age).

SECTION II

PUTTING THE NUTRITIONAL PIECES TOGETHER IN THE BACKCOUNTRY

Food is our common ground, a universal experience.
—James Beard

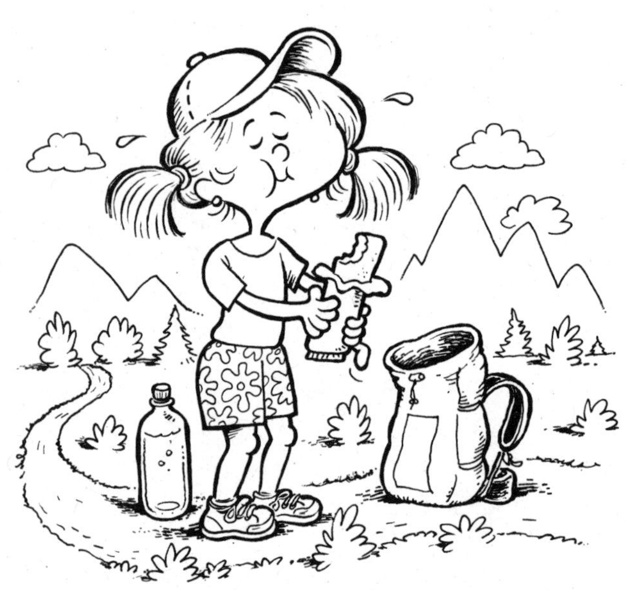

Now that you have a solid nutritional foundation from the backcountry nutrition basics in section I, you are ready to learn how these concepts are more specifically applied in the field. In the quest to go beyond mere backcountry survival, chapter 7 at the beginning of this section will discuss food and mood. While some of the connections may be obvious, such as being hungry can make you cranky, others are not obvious at all, like the fact that eating carbohydrates increases the amount of tryptophan that gets into your brain to make serotonin, the brain chemical that makes you feel calm. This chapter also discusses coffee, chocolate, food cravings, and food shortages in the field.

In chapter 8, you will learn ways to keep your immune system strong, as well as what to do nutritionally when backcountry illness strikes. Chapter 9 addresses nutritional considerations for special environments, such as extreme cold, heat, and high altitude, which can all significantly impact your nutritional needs and your ability to meet these needs.

The information in chapter 10 is for young backcountry travelers, who are essentially eating for growth and development. Despite potentially higher requirements for certain nutrients, teens may not consider nutrition a priority in the backcountry; therefore, they need nutrition information in order to understand that *what* they eat affects everyday short-term performance (moods, energy levels, and muscle building).

One of the challenges of backcountry nutrition is making some nutritional tradeoffs to accommodate unique diets and the limited resources for food storage and preservation, while getting the nutrients you need for optimal health and performance. If you have special dietary concerns, chapter 11 addresses some of the nutritional considerations related to vegetarian diets, food allergy, and food intolerance. Chapter 12 discusses the transition from field to home and the nutritional habits you may want to take home with you, as well as those habits best left in the backcountry. This and chapter 13, devoted to the backcountry professional, are important for those of you who choose to live and work in the field for much of the year.

CHAPTER 7

FOOD AND MOOD

Each night one recipe was read from a cookbook they had salvaged. "This would be discussed very seriously," Shackleton wrote, "and alterations and improvements suggested, and then they would turn into their [sleeping] bags to dream of wonderful meals that they could never reach."

—Ernest Shackleton's Diary

While calories and water are backcountry essentials, it is useful to understand how nutrition can take you beyond survival and into enjoyment of your backcountry adventure and some of the less obvious ways nutrition affects your backcountry experience. The food and mood connection was introduced in the carbohydrate chapter with respect to blood sugar levels. Low blood sugar can dramatically affect your energy levels, coordination and balance, ability to think clearly, and your mood. The way you interact with your group in the backcountry can make the difference between an enjoyable experience and a difficult one. In fact, group dynamics can affect the overall success of an expedition.

This doesn't mean that a few crabby moments will ruin the trip for everyone. However, there are plenty of stressful situations that arise in the backcountry that can cause moods to plummet and tempers to flare. Many of these situations are beyond your control and you will just need to make the best of them. It makes sense, however, to head off the stressors that you can prevent, like low blood sugar and dehydration from inadequate fuel and water.

> ► **Chocolate is a comfort food for many backcountry travelers. Look for varieties in a special wax package that prevents melting.**

In addition to low blood sugar and dehydration, a variety of nutrients are needed to make hormones and other brain chemicals that affect your mood

Brain Chemicals Related to Food and Mood

Neurotransmitters:

Serotonin

- Regulates sleep, mood, food intake, pain tolerance
- Low levels related to insomnia, depression, food cravings (especially carbs), increased sensitivity to pain, aggressive behavior, and poor body temperature regulation
- Made from the amino acid tryptophan (Trp)
- Requires vitamins B_6, B_{12}, and folic acid to convert from Trp
- A protein-rich meal decreases serotonin levels (large amino acids compete to get to the brain)
- A carbohydrate-rich meal causes insulin secretion and increases serotonin levels in brain.

Dopamine and Norepinephrine

- Decreased levels of these are associated with depression and mood disorders
- Made from the amino acid tyrosine (Tyr)
- Production requires vitamin B_{12}, folic acid, magnesium; norepinephrine also requires vitamin C
- A high-protein meal favors Tyr production
- Those who do not respond to a high-carbohydrate meal for improved mood may benefit from a high-protein meal to increase dopamine and norepinephrine levels.

Neuropeptide Y, Galanin, Endorphins

- Stimulate appetite and increase our desire to eat.

Cholecystokinin

- Works in small intestine, sends satiety signals to brain.

Other Brain Chemicals

Endorphins: opioids related to "feeling good" (one reason we crave sweet foods and exercise).

Choline: fatlike substance used in cell membranes; important for memory and mental functioning; occurs in food as part of lecithin.

Essential Fatty Acids (EFAs): component of cell membranes, especially in the brain and eyes.

and ability to think. You may be familiar with the neurotransmitter serotonin that is involved in depression and other mood disorders. To make and use serotonin, your body needs the amino acid tryptophan (found in protein foods), along with a release of insulin from eating carbohydrates, to usher the tryptophan into your brain. You also need vitamins B_6, B_{12}, and folate for this process to run smoothly.

Without getting too technical, the point is that nutrition is related to every aspect of your health, including your mental health. The previous table includes some of the brain chemicals that affect mood and appetite, and the next table includes a variety of nutrients that are needed to make and use these various compounds. You will see that many of the food sources of these important nutrients are easily taken into the backcountry. Once again, getting enough calories from a variety of foods is your best chance of meeting all of your nutrient needs in the backcountry. However, there is a caveat: you then have to time your meals and snacks so that you get the food and water when you need them in order to keep blood sugar levels steady and your cells well hydrated.

Food Sources of Nutrients Related to Mood

Nutrient	***Food Sources***
B vitamins and vitamins C and E are needed to make neurotransmitters (brain chemicals) such as serotonin, dopamine, and norepinephrine	
Vitamin B_1 (thiamin)	Wheat germ, greens, oranges, legumes, nutritional yeast, whole grain bread, sunflower seeds
Vitamin B_2 (riboflavin)	Milk, yogurt, avocado, spinach, broccoli, whole grain bread, cheese, mushrooms
Vitamin B_3 (niacin)	Meat/chicken/fish, peanut butter, potatoes, brewer's yeast, wheat germ, yogurt, mushrooms

Vitamin B_6 (pyridoxine)	Bananas, avocados, meat/chicken/fish, nutritional yeast, wheat germ, sunflower seeds, potatoes, collard greens, black beans, peanut butter, almonds, walnuts, hazelnuts
Vitamin B_{12} (cobalamin)	Tuna, oysters, yogurt, milk, fish, chicken, cheese, fortified foods
Pantothenic Acid	Oranges, collard greens, potatoes, broccoli, brown rice, cantaloupe, wheat germ, salmon, chicken, yogurt, sweet potatoes, eggs
Biotin	Oatmeal, soybeans, peanut butter, salmon, milk, brown rice, chicken, eggs, wheat germ
Folic Acid	Nutritional yeast, spinach (and other leafy greens), oranges, avocados, broccoli, wheat germ, legumes, bananas, whole wheat bread
Vitamin C	Papaya, bell and chili peppers, citrus fruit, broccoli, strawberries, collards, kale, peas, potatoes, yam, squash, tomato, melon
Vitamin E	Vegetable and nut oils, whole grains, wheat germ, sunflower seeds, sesame seeds, almonds, soybeans
The following minerals help convert amino acids from protein foods into brain chemicals (neurotransmitters and hormones)	
Magnesium (mineral) Also protects neurotransmitters from damage	Peanuts, bananas, milk, wheat germ, spinach, whole wheat bread, pecans, cruciferous vegetables (broccoli, cabbage, etc.), beans, lentils, chocolate
Iron (mineral) Also aids neurotransmitter activity	Spinach, kale, meat, legumes, apricots, raisins, pumpkin seeds, whole wheat bread, nuts

Food Sources of Nutrients Related to Mood (continued)

Nutrient	*Food Sources*
Calcium	Yogurt, milk, many soy products, black strap molasses, figs, almonds, sesame seeds
Lipids (fats and fatlike substances): used to make and protect cell membranes of brain chemicals	
Essential Fatty Acids (omega-3 fats)	Cold-water fish (salmon, tuna, herring, etc.), walnuts, soybeans, flaxseeds
Choline/lecithin (fatlike substance)	Egg yolk, peanuts, wheat germ, soybeans, brewer's yeast

This is not an exhaustive list; there are many other nutrients that play roles in the production of brain chemicals. Copyright Beyond Broccoli Nutrition Counseling.

CAFFEINE IN THE BACKCOUNTRY

Without my morning coffee, I'm just like a dried up piece of roast goat.
—Johann Sebastian Bach (1685–1750), *The Coffee Cantata*

A discussion about food and mood would not be complete without mentioning caffeine. The effects of caffeine vary from person to person and for regular users, but the effects on mood are generally uplifting. As a central nervous system stimulant, caffeine can increase your ability to focus and help you feel more energetic. Overuse of caffeine can backfire, however, causing the jitters, irritability, anxiety, diarrhea, and insomnia. In fact, for nonusers or people sensitive to caffeine, these effects may occur with a small amount. Insomnia, irritability, and headaches are also caffeine-withdrawal symptoms that can occur if a regular user gets less caffeine than usual.

Studies have linked caffeine use to sleep problems, migraine headaches, Premenstrual Syndrome (PMS) symptoms, low-birthweight babies (consumption during pregnancy), and it may exacerbate high blood pressure and irregular heart rhythms. Caffeine may also irritate the bowel and increase symptoms of gastroesophageal reflux disease (GERD) and gout (a type of arthritis). Several years ago it was thought that drinking coffee increased the risk of pancreatic cancer, but this has since been debunked; smoking turned out to be the real culprit, and many smokers also happen to drink coffee.

> **did you know ?**
>
> Food choices are driven by both the need for calories and the desire for pleasure.

If you are accustomed to drinking a fair amount of caffeine in the front-country (coffee, tea, carbonated beverages) you may want to consider a transition plan before venturing into the backcountry. If you plan to consume less caffeine than usual (many outdoor programs such as NOLS don't issue coffee), you could wean yourself prior to your trip to prevent the unpleasant effects of withdrawal. On the other hand, packing tea bags or instant coffee takes up little room in your pack and may make a transition from several cups a day to one or two somewhat easier. You don't have to completely forego caffeine in the field. However, decreasing your dependence on caffeine will keep the probable side effects (like irritability) at bay, particularly at the beginning of your journey when your body is building muscle and adjusting to a field diet that may vary significantly from your frontcountry fare.

Another concern with caffeine in the backcountry is its ability to interfere with iron absorption and to leach calcium from your bones. While caffeine consumption can promote calcium losses, at least one study found that the losses were balanced later in the day with increased absorption. If, however, you are eating a vegetarian field diet that relies on the less well-absorbed plant sources of iron (nonheme), you may want to drink caffeinated beverages between meals (see the vitamin chapter in section I or the special diet chapter in this section for more information about iron sources). Or you may choose to forego caffeine in the backcountry altogether.

On a positive note, one high-altitude study showed that tea (with caffeine) did not negatively affect hydration status, and it improved mood and reduced the perception of fatigue. If you enjoy a cup of hot tea at camp and it doesn't interfere with your sleep, this may be another way to increase your fluid intake on cold days. Also, three of the most popular caffeine delivery systems, coffee, tea (black, green, and oolong), and chocolate, contain

Caffeine Content of Backcountry Foods and Beverages

Food/Beverage	*Serving Size*	*Amount of Caffeine (mg)*
*Coffee, instant	5 oz.	60 to 80
Decaffeinated coffee	5 oz.	1 to 5
Espresso	2 oz.	40 to 170
*Tea, brewed	5 oz.	20 to 110
Tea, instant	5 oz.	25 to 50
Milk chocolate	1 oz.	1 to 15
Dark chocolate	1 oz.	5 to 35
Baker's chocolate	1 oz.	25

*Amount of caffeine varies with brewing time and process (French press, cone filter, percolator, etc.).

> ► **Make your own cocoa with added calcium and protein, the amount of sweetness you enjoy, and no trans fat. Mix unsweetened cocoa powder, powdered milk, sugar, and ground cinnamon.**

powerful antioxidant compounds that may be beneficial in the backcountry (see chapter 6 for more about antioxidants).

In addition to positive or negative effects on mood, caffeine is credited with significant performance-enhancing properties for endurance sports. It may reduce the fatigue that comes with long periods of exercise and enhance muscle strength at the end of a long day on the trail. The still touted diuretic effects of caffeine are now considered minor, and in many athletes (especially habituated caffeine users) nonexistent. In 2004 the World Anti-Doping Association and the International Olympic Committee removed caffeine from its banned substances list, though the National Collegiate Athletic Association still restricts urine levels of caffeine for young athletes. Though a debate continues in the athletic community about this decision, it suggests that caffeine may be used safely among athletes. The effects of caffeine also vary according to tolerance, and some evidence suggests regular caffeine users do not experience the boost in sports performance that

> **did you know ?**
>
> Research shows that stress can cause you to crave palatable or comfort foods *and* eating these foods can affect how your body responds to both physiological and psychological stress.

Chocolate in the Backcountry

The effects of chocolate on mood may depend upon the amount and type consumed (white chocolate is not real chocolate) and differs from person to person. It is also difficult to know how much of the love affair with chocolate is cultural (it is used so often for gifts, rewards, and treats) and how much is physiological. According to Elizabeth Somer, author of the book *Food & Mood*, chocolate does affect almost every appetite-stimulating brain chemical and has many effects on mood.

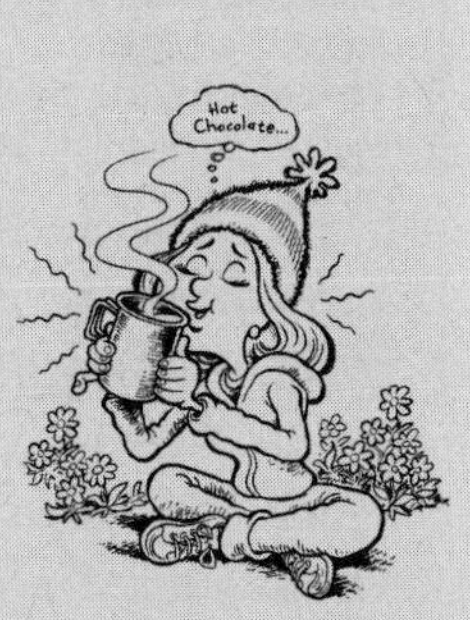

Here are some ways chocolate may affect mood:

- Chocolate stimulates release of the brain chemical serotonin (calming effect).
- Cocoa butter, a component of real chocolate, is solid at room temperature and melts at body temperature, resulting in a pleasurable texture or "mouthfeel."
- Theobromine and caffeine in chocolate provide a mental lift.
- The combination of sugar, fat, and PEA (phenylethylamine) in chocolate stimulates an endorphin (chemical related to pleasure) release in the brain.
- PEA also stimulates the nervous system and increases blood pressure and heart rate, simulating the feelings experienced when "in love." (Note: PEA is also in cheese and salami—foods not known for this effect!)

Given the real potential advantages of comfort foods in dealing with stress, if chocolate (especially dark chocolate) happens to be one of your comfort foods, it could be a welcome addition to your backcountry menu.

nonusers do, unless they take a break from it prior to using it to enhance performance.

FOOD PSYCHOLOGY

I have had very few food cravings, although last night I dreamt I was stuffing myself with sweet potatoes and I don't even like sweet potatoes.
—Appalachian Trail Hiker

Nutrition goes beyond the hard facts related to various nutrients and how they affect your body. There is a tendency among hard-

► **One small dark chocolate candy bar (1 to 2 ounces) has roughly the same amount of the phytonutrient antioxidants as a 5-ounce glass of red wine.**

core backcountry users to dismiss the less quantifiable aspects of nutrition for a desire to just stick to the basics. Bring food (for calories) and water. Again, this gets back to the premise of this book, which is to go beyond mere survival. It may be helpful to understand a few things about how we think about food and why we may react the way we do to situations such as food shortages in the backcountry. It may also help to know that comfort foods can actually help your body respond to both physiological and psychological stress. Finally, food cravings may mean that you need more carbohydrates for energy, or it may simply be a response to a limited menu and not an indication that you are suffering from a nutrient deficiency.

There are many reasons we eat and many factors that play a role in which foods we choose, how much we eat, and how we feel throughout the whole eating process. Inevitably, many backcountry groups end up talking about food a lot, especially on longer trips. Given the simplicity of backcountry living compared to our everyday lives, this makes sense. In the backcountry you are literally back to a more basic level of existence. Food, water, shelter, clothing, and human-powered transportation are the focus, along with whatever goals you have for your backcountry journey.

Meals are an important part of community in the backcountry, a time to share experiences from the day's journey and to plan for the next day. While some people just want a meal at the end of the day and don't care much what it is, others use cooking and food preparation as a creative outlet or an opportunity to create their backcountry version of comfort food. In some outdoor education programs like NOLS, learning to cook is an integral part of the program. If you know how to feed yourself well, you are more likely to survive, and thrive, in the backcountry.

did you know?

Unusual meals or meals that don't meet your expectations, in composition or size, can negatively affect your mood.

FOOD-RELATED STRESS

I went through U.S. Army Ranger School so my perceptions of "going hungry" or best/worst foods are warped. If it isn't an MRE I'm happy!
—Appalachian Trail Hiker

"Not long ago I ate a whole chicken, a calzone, and a 12-cut pizza and although I could not physically eat more, I was still hungry. At every road crossing I have to force myself not to run for food. I dream about food. For fun I go to supermarkets and look at food. My last through hike in '98 I lost 40 pounds."
—Appalachian Trail Through-Hiker

Food shortages can pose significant psychological and physiological challenges in the backcountry. Sometimes taking bare minimum rations is intentional to save weight or pack space or to allow faster travel. If the whole group is involved in the decision to travel this way, the rations are carefully planned, and perhaps at least some of the group members have experience with this type of expedition, it may be a very satisfying experience with few or no negative effects.

If, however, the group does not expect lighter rations or an unplanned event leads to a food shortage (losing a cache to avalanche, animals, poor navigation, or missing a re-ration pick up), many of the psychological (and physiological) consequences of food deprivation may set in. The severity of the shortage and length of time involved will also determine how the group reacts.

The physiological effects of a food shortage (or a forced fasting situation) are starvation responses that include lethargy, fatigue, stomach pain, and acetone breath (from the ketone compounds produced when your body breaks down muscle for fuel). In fact, when you continue to exercise while not providing your body with adequate fuel, your body will produce toxins as it breaks down protein and fat for glu-

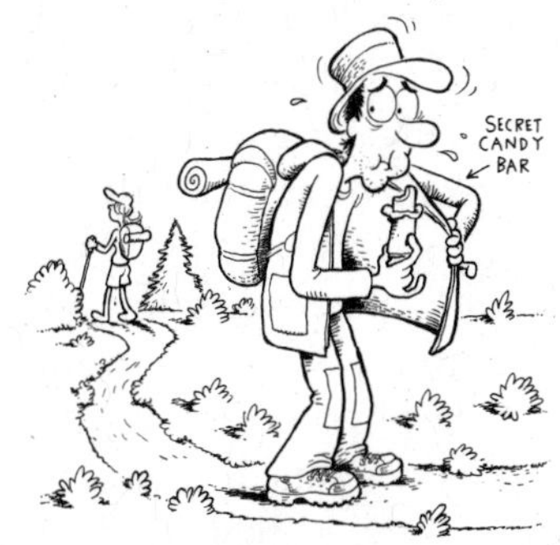

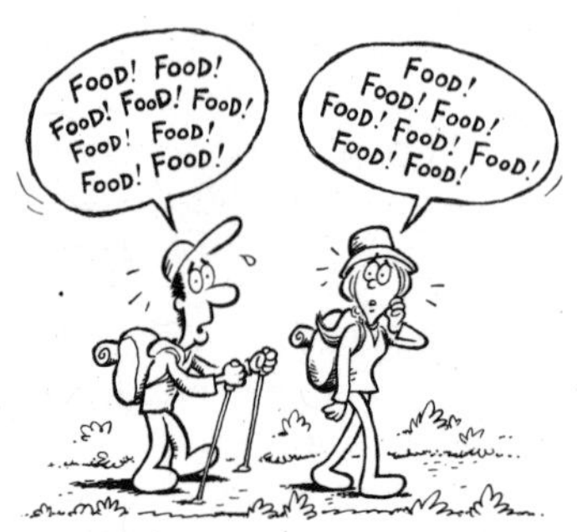

cose. Your digestive system "rests," since it has no food to process, but this also slows down your overall metabolism to preserve its energy stores.

If you do find yourself in this situation, it is essential to your survival that you maintain adequate water and electrolyte intake. In fact, it is best to actually increase your water intake if you do not have food, since your body relies on the water that it gets from food (both the water in the food and the water produced during digestion) to fuel metabolic processes. Electrolytes, especially salt, are also critical to prevent some of the physiological imbalances that occur when losses through sweat and respiration are not replaced with food and drink.

Some of the psychological reactions to food deprivation include a preoccupation with food and eating, increased distractibility, restlessness, malaise, increased emotional responses, and when food becomes available again, binge eating and hoarding food. Another interesting phenomenon may be related to the fact that we live in a culture that has virtually unlimited access to a wide variety of foods. If you perceive that your amounts or types of food choices are limited, you may experience some of the same psychological effects that a true food shortage evokes. The seemingly endless discussions about food and eating in the backcountry that was mentioned above may actually be part of this. Food cravings may also be linked to this sense of deprivation. While these effects are not generally long term, some backcountry travelers do notice a lingering desire for certain foods after returning home.

There is no consensus among nutrition professionals regarding the reasons for food cravings. While some cravings directly correlate to physiological needs, like craving salty foods during or after strenuous activity that leads to sodium

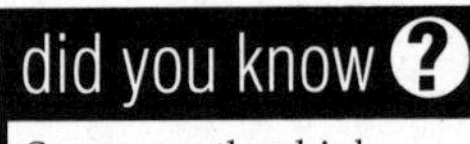

Sweet or other high-calorie foods can improve your mood.

losses or carbohydrates when blood sugar is low, other desires are less clear. If you are eating enough calories, including foods rich in carbohydrate, fat, and protein, cravings are likely to be psychologically or emotionally based. This does not make them any less real or any less important, given the research that supports the role of comfort foods in helping your body respond to stress.

Ideally, in addition to the nutritional considerations related to physical health and performance, ration planning should take all of these psychological factors into account as well. The NOLS rations are an excellent example of a well-rounded backcountry pantry. The trail foods include a combination of tastes and textures (sweet, salty, chewy, and crunchy), varied at each re-ration to keep it interesting. The spice kit is a key component of every ration, and there are desserts and basic items needed for backcountry baking. (I have vivid memories of baking pizza on a rest day in the Absaroka Wilderness on my NOLS course.)

So, in addition to your food choices for optimal nutrition to fuel yourself in the backcountry, remember to take along some of your favorite treat foods that pack well and may be a hard-earned reward at the end of a tough backcountry day.

CHAPTER 8 STAYING HEALTHY AND MANAGING ILLNESS

Those who think they have no time for healthy eating will sooner or later have to find time for illness."
—modified from Edward Stanley (1826–1893), *The Conduct of Life*

KEEPING YOUR IMMUNE SYSTEM STRONG

While staying healthy is not a goal reserved for the backcountry, most would agree that being sick in the comfort of your home is significantly better than being sick in a tent in some remote area. In addition to discomfort, losing excessive nutrients and fluid due to diarrhea and/or vomiting can lead to electrolyte imbalances, dehydration, and fatigue that delay recovery, which is especially detrimental and challenging if you are part of a group that needs to keep moving. There are some nutritional strategies that can keep your immune system strong and others to help you manage and recover from illness in the backcountry.

DRINK ENOUGH FLUID

You need a minimum of 3 to 4 liters per day. Dehydration makes every system in your body work harder—including your immune system. If you don't drink enough on one day, you need to drink more than usual the next day to "catch up" since dehydration is cumulative. Make sure your urine is light yellow to clear and that you are urinating often. To make sure your body can absorb what you drink, take in small amounts of fluid throughout the day rather than large amounts periodically.

EAT ENOUGH CALORIES

This could be anywhere from 2,500 to 5,000 per day, or more. Getting enough fuel in the backcountry from a variety of foods will help you get enough of the various nutrients your body's immune system needs to work well.

EAT ENOUGH CARBOHYDRATES

Aim for 3.6 to 4.5 grams per pound (8 to 10 grams per kilogram) of body weight per day. Exercising with depleted glycogen (carbohydrate) stores increases your risk of injury. Low blood sugar also can decrease immunity, so eating carbs throughout the day to maintain blood sugar levels is also important.

EAT ENOUGH PROTEIN

Eat .6 to .9 grams per pound (1.3 to 2.0 grams per kilogram) of body weight per day. Antibodies and other important immune system compounds are made from the amino acids your body gets from the protein you eat. You cannot store protein, so you need to eat it every day. If your body doesn't meet its protein needs from food, then it will break down muscle for amino acids. Enough protein is important, but excess protein does not help your immune system, requires more water to process, and actually can make your kidneys work harder.

EAT ENOUGH FAT

Fats should make up 20 to 35 percent of your total calories. Fat is also important for your immune system, especially omega-3 and omega-6, the essential fatty acids. The latest recommendations suggest that 10 percent of your fat intake should be from these beneficial fats found in fish and various plant foods.

EAT A VARIETY OF FOODS

Eating a variety of foods (assuming at least that some are nutritious) will help you get the vitamins, minerals, and phytonutrients that your immune system needs to work well. Omitting whole food groups is not a good idea unless you have an allergy, intolerance, or food preferences, and have adjusted your field diet to fill in any nutritional gaps.

► **As boring as it may sound, washing your hands and treating your water are probably the most important habits to keep you from getting ill in the backcountry.**

NUTRITION AND BACKCOUNTRY ILLNESS

FOOD-BORNE ILLNESS

It is estimated that many cases of the twenty-four-hour flu are in fact related to viruses that spread from contaminated and/or improperly handled food or water. In the backcountry, hygiene is very important. Wash your hands with soap after defecating and prior to preparing or eating food. Unless you are traveling in the winter and can keep foods out of the danger zone for bacterial growth (40°F to 140°F), saving leftovers from dinner to eat the following day is not a good idea. If you can keep leftovers from dinner cold at night and heat it thoroughly the next morning, it may be an acceptable breakfast option, but putting cooked food in a pack and eating it several hours later is not safe.

This recommendation is difficult for some avid backpackers and climbers to accept since many of us (yes, I am included in this one) have personal experience with saving dinner leftovers for lunch the next day, or perhaps even dinner the next evening. One AT hiker commented that cooked burger will last two days on the trail and "makes a great additive for the evening gruel." Each of us has a different tolerance to pathogens, and if your immune system is strong, you may be able to tolerate more than another member of your group can. It is also possible that some of the herbs and spices used to prepare food can help keep food safe (this is one of the reasons many cultures began using spices in food preparation). Unfortunately, we don't know which spices or the amount needed to consistently keep food safe. If you boast what my mom used to call "a cast-iron stomach," (as the AT hiker I quoted appears to) you may be able to get away with sloppy food handling, but you need to know there are risks.

The following table lists common food-borne pathogens, how they are transmitted, their symptoms, and some guidelines for dealing with diarrhea, nausea, and vomiting that can result from contaminated food or water.

Bacteria that Cause Food-borne Illness

Bacteria	*Found*	*Transmission*	*Symptoms*
Campylobacter jejuni	Intestinal tracts of animals and birds	Contaminated water, raw milk, raw or undercooked meat, untreated poultry, shellfish water, sewage sludge	Fever, headache and muscle pain followed by diarrhea (sometimes bloody), abdominal pain, and nausea that appear 2 to 5 days after eating; may last 7 to 10 days
Clostridium botulinum	Widely distributed in nature: soil, water, plants, and intestinal tracts of animals and fish; grows only in little or no oxygen; produces a toxin that causes illness	Improperly canned foods, garlic in oil, vacuum-packed and tightly wrapped food	Toxin affects the nervous system; symptoms usually appear after 18 to 36 hours, but can sometimes appear as few as 4 hours or as many as 8 days after eating: double vision, droopy eyelids, trouble speaking and swallowing, difficulty breathing; fatal in 3 to 10 days if not treated
Clostridium perfringens	Soil, dust, sewage, and intestinal tracts of animals and humans; grows only in little or no oxygen	Called "the cafeteria germ" because many outbreaks result from food left for long periods in steam tables or at room temperature; bacteria destroyed by cooking, but some toxin-producing spores may survive	Diarrhea and gas pains may appear 8 to 24 hours after eating; usually last about 1 day, but less severe symptoms may persist for 1 to 2 weeks

Bacteria that Cause Food-borne Illness (continued)			
Escherichia coli 0157:H7	Intestinal tracts of some mammals, raw milk, unchlorinated water; one of several strains of E. coli that can cause human illness	Contaminated water, raw milk, raw or rare ground beef, unpasteurized apple juice or cider, uncooked fruits and vegetables; person to person, especially the very young	Diarrhea or bloody diarrhea, abdominal cramps, nausea, and malaise; can begin 2 to 5 days after food is eaten, lasting about 8 days; some, have developed hemolytic-uremic syndrome (HUS) that causes acute kidney failure
Listeria monocytogenes	Intestinal tracts of humans and animals, milk, soil, leaf vegvetables; can grow slowly at refrigerator temperatures	Ready-to-eat foods such as hot dogs, luncheon meats, cold cuts, fermented or dry sausage, and other deli-style meat and poultry, soft cheeses and unpasteurized milk	Fever, chills, headache, backache, sometimes upset stomach, abdominal pain and diarrhea; may take up to 3 weeks to become ill; may later develop more serious illness in at-risk patients (pregnant women and newborns, older adults, and people with weakened immune systems)

Salmonella (over 2,300 types)	Intestinal tracts and feces of animals; Salmonella Enteritidis in eggs	Raw or undercooked eggs, poultry, and meat; raw milk and dairy products; seafood; food handlers	Stomach pain, diarrhea, nausea, chills, fever, and headache usually appear 8 to 72 hours after eating; may last 1 to 2 days
Shigella (over 30 types)	Human intestinal tract; rarely found in other animals	Person to person by fecal-oral route; fecal contamination of food and water. Most outbreaks result from food, especially salads, prepared and handled by workers using poor personal hygiene	Disease referred to as "shigellosis" or bacillary dysentery; diarrhea containing blood and mucus, fever, abdominal cramps, chills, and vomiting; 12 to 50 hours from ingestion of bacteria; can last a few days to 2 weeks
Staphylococcus aureus	On humans (skin, infected cuts, pimples, noses, and throats)	Person to person through food from improper food handling; multiply rapidly at room temperature to produce a toxin that causes illness	Severe nausea, abdominal cramps, vomiting, and diarrhea occur 1 to 6 hours after eating; recovery within 2 to 3 days, longer if severe dehydration occurs

www.fsis.usda.gov/Fact_Sheets/Foodborne_Illness_What_Consumers_Need_to_Know/index.asp (Last Modified: April 3, 2006)

DIARRHEA

According to a study of long-distance hikers published in 2003, diarrhea is the most common illness limiting long-distance hiking. In fact, this is true of nearly every study of hikers, trekkers, and expeditions and is true for NOLS courses. There are many causes of diarrhea in the backcountry, such as contaminated food, water, a virus, food intolerance, or other unknown reasons. Fecal matter on hands and contaminated water are two risks that can be minimized by proper backcountry hygiene (hand washing) and disinfecting all water used for eating, drinking, and cleaning dishes. If untreated water is used to clean dishes, the dishes should be left to dry completely, preferably in the sun, before using them again.

Irregular bowel movements are common while adjusting to a new environment. Diarrhea is an increase in frequency of bowel movements compared to usual patterns, or excess water content of stool that affects consistency, volume, or both. If it is accompanied by bloating and excessive intestinal gas, it may be a response to an excessive amount of fructose (too much dried fruit or drink mixes that contain high fructose corn syrup) or other food intolerance.

While many foods that pose a high risk for contamination are fresh foods that are not commonly eaten in the backcountry, it is still important to consider basic food safety in terms of washing your hands after urinating and defecating and before preparing food or eating. *Diarrhea can be a very serious issue in the backcountry because of its link to dehydration.*

Treatment strategies for diarrhea

Drink plenty of clear liquids (properly treated water, noncaffeinated tea, and broth). Include beverages and soft foods with salt to replace losses (broth and hot cereal with added salt). Avoid raw fruits and vegetables, whole grains, coffee, spices, alcohol, and concentrated sweets

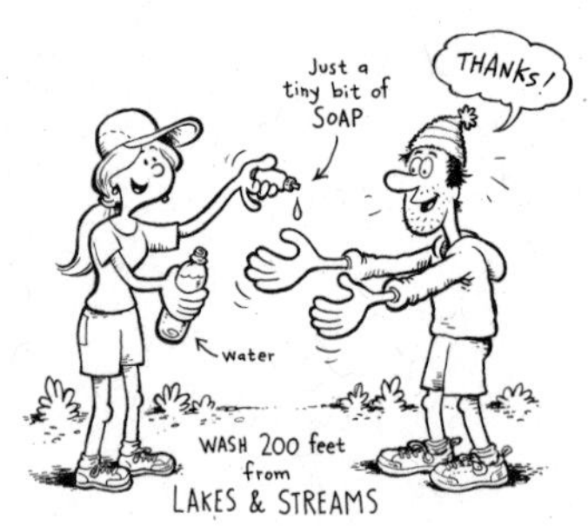
Just a tiny bit of SOAP
THANKS!
Water
WASH 200 feet from LAKES & STREAMS

(dried fruit, candy, and sweet drink mix) until the diarrhea stops. Eat small meals throughout the day, which may be tolerated better than a few large meals.

If diarrhea continues for more than a day or you are experiencing symptoms of dehydration, prepare an ORS (oral rehydrating solution) to correct imbalances of both fluid and electrolytes. If your medical kit does not have a prepared ORS, the World Health Organization recommends mixing 6 teaspoons of sugar, 1 teaspoon of salt, and one liter of treated water.

CONSTIPATION

Another common gastrointestinal problem is constipation. The definition of "normal" with respect to elimination of waste is somewhat controversial. Most gastroenterologists consider normal ranges for bowel movements to be anywhere from 3 to 21 times per week. Some people go even less than that with no ill effects. What matters more than the frequency is how things pass: hard stools, the need to strain to eliminate, and a feeling that elimination isn't complete afterwards are considered abnormal.

Changes in diet, both what you eat and your pattern of eating, exercise, the stress associated with travel, and not enough fluid are all common causes of constipation in the backcountry. For some it takes two to three days for the bowels to adjust to backcountry living. Others never really adjust well.

Fiber and fluid are the key to remaining regular. Getting enough dietary fiber is typically not a problem in the backcountry since grains, nuts, seeds, dried fruit, and other foods high in fiber are commonly eaten. The part many people don't understand is that fiber must be combined with enough fluids to have a laxative effect. We've already established that in the backcountry the high level of physical activity often combined with dry, hot, cold, or high-altitude environments make getting enough fluid a major challenge. If your frontcountry diet is not typically as high in fiber as your backcountry diet, you now have another factor that increases your water needs.

For some individuals, milk, nuts, cheese, chocolate, and an excessive amount of refined carbohydrates (white bread, rice, pasta, etc.) can contribute to constipation. Since some of these foods (nuts, milk, cheese, etc.) are important in the backcountry for balanced nutrition and convenience (refined grains cook fast, are light-weight, and last longer) getting more fluid is the best first step if you are not comfortable with your bowel schedule.

Habits that can help relieve constipation

Drink water first thing upon waking. Some people find warm or hot water works better than cold water to get things moving. Get up and move around a bit before breakfast; exercise can stimulate the bowels. Use relaxation techniques such as deep breathing or meditation if you are feeling stress about the fact that your bowel movements are not normal.

Probiotics

One popular nutritional approach to several gastrointestinal problems is the use of probiotic foods and supplements. Probiotic, as contrasted to antibiotic, means "for life" and refers to the colonies of beneficial bacteria that live in the gastrointestinal (GI) tract. These "good bugs" help keep the harmful bacteria at bay and have shown promise in strengthening immunity in a variety of ways, in addition to helping GI issues such as diarrhea, bloating, and constipation. There is even some research that suggests probiotics may help with food allergies: if a "leaky gut" has allowed proteins to leave the intestines and enter the bloodstream, probiotics may help strengthen the intestinal walls and prevent this leakage.

There are many different strains of probiotics and only a handful of these strains have been well studied. One of the problems with both probiotic foods and supplements is the ability for the bacteria to survive the trip through the highly acidic stomach before getting to the intestines where they do their work. While food sources don't tend to start with as many bacteria as supplements, components in food may help the bacteria get through the stomach intact. On the other hand, supplements begin with higher levels of probiotics, knowing only a certain percentage are likely to survive digestion, and this is often the preferred way to recolonize the GI tract following a course of antibiotics.

The most common probiotic foods, such as yogurt, kefir, and special beverages, are not suitable for backcountry travel. There are, however, some energy-type bars and cereals that have added probiotics, as well as shelf-stable supplements (they do not need to be refrigerated). If you know you have a sensitive digestive system and are prone to diarrhea and/or constipation, it may be worth packing some of these foods or supplements. The general thinking at this time is that you need to get a consistent supply of the probiotics (eat probiotic foods or take the pills daily) to address specific issues such as diarrhea. Luckily many common backcountry foods high in fiber act as "prebiotics" to feed the probiotics and help increase their numbers naturally.

The August 2007 issue of *Environmental Nutrition Newsletter* published the following guidelines for buying probiotics:

- In foods look for *Lactobacillus* or *Bifidobacterium.*
- Some foods that have evidence to show they survive the GI tract and increase the good bacteria that may be taken into the backcountry include Attune wellness bars and Kashi Vive cereal. (Note from the website for the Attune bars: "We ship and sell Attune wellness bars refrigerated to keep the probiotics effective for the maximum amount of time. However, our unique formulation and robust probiotics remain alive at sufficient levels without refrigeration at normal ambient temperatures for up to three months.")
- In supplements look for at least four to ten billion Colony Forming Units (CFU) per dose.
- Some of the brands that have been tested by ConsumerLab.com and live up to their label claims: Nature's Way *Primadophilus* Optima 14 Probiotic Strain Plus NutraFlora, Jarrow Formulas Enhanced Probiotic system Jarro-Dophilus PS, Kyo-Dophilus, and Probiotic Gut Buddies. Dr. Andrew Weil also recommends supplements with the *Lactobacillus* GG, and one brand that contains this strain is Culturelle.
- If you are traveling to an undeveloped area where the water supply is questionable prior to beginning your backcountry adventure, it may be helpful to take a probiotic supplement prior to and during the time you will be exposed to potentially harmful bacteria that can cause traveler's diarrhea. Though there is not a lot of solid research to support the benefits, many people who travel extensively are convinced probiotics can help.

NAUSEA AND VOMITING

Nausea and vomiting may be related to illness caused by either bacteria or viruses in the backcountry. Nausea is the sensation that you need to vomit and may occur with or without actual vomiting. Nausea can be related to low blood sugar, motion sickness, pregnancy, or vertigo that results from injury. Mild nausea may be treated with ginger tea or candied ginger, dry foods such as crackers, toast or cereal, or tart foods. Cold foods or other foods that have little or no odor may be better tolerated. Relaxing, chewing foods well, breathing deeply, and sipping beverages other than plain water may also help nausea.

Vomiting (getting rid of gastrointestinal contents) often follows sweating, salivation, dilated pupils, pallor, and sometimes wretching. Like diarrhea, one of the consequences of vomiting in the backcountry is dehydration and electrolyte depletion, but many other nutrients are also lost. Obviously, the longer that vomiting lasts the more dangerous it becomes. Depending on the amount of food one is able to tolerate after vomiting, muscle and overall weakness, fatigue, and dizziness are likely to occur.

> ► **Drink more fluid if you are sick and cannot eat.**

Nutritional approaches to treat vomiting

Eat small, frequent meals. Eat quickly digested and absorbed foods (crackers, white rice, white breads, low-fiber cereals) between bouts. Sip liquids between meals rather than with meals. Cold liquids may be better tolerated than hot liquids. Avoid strong-flavored foods, coffee, high-fat foods (especially fried), and whole milk (skim milk may be okay for some people). Avoid highly acidic foods. Rest for at least an hour following meals. Eat whatever will stay with you. (This varies and may even include some foods from the "don't" list!)

DEHYDRATION

Chapter 2 includes detailed information about water's nutritional role and how much we need, but dehydration appears again in this chapter because water is such an important nutrient. Though you don't get energy from water per se, every cell in your body needs water to work well. Also, you need to keep up with your fluid needs every day. If you are slightly dehydrated one day, you will begin the next day at a deficit and need more fluid to bring your hydration into balance again. Another important point is that you don't experience thirst during exercise until you are already dehydrated, so it is important to begin drinking before you are thirsty.

> **did you know ?**
>
> Cold fluids leave your stomach faster and are absorbed more quickly than room temperature liquids.

Your urine and bowel movements are a good way to assess whether or not you are drinking enough fluid. Urine should be straw colored or clear

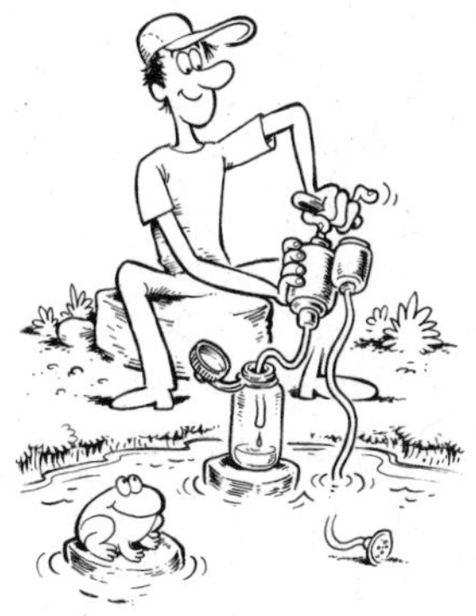

(unless you just took a vitamin supplement; riboflavin will make urine dark), and you should pee often if you are properly hydrating throughout the day. If you are adjusting to high altitude or are suddenly exposed to cold temperatures, you may urinate excessively (altitude- or cold-induced diuresis), but this does not mean you are adequately hydrated. In fact, these environments can make it more difficult both to get enough fluid and then to stay hydrated. Hard, dry stools that are difficult to pass can be a symptom of inadequate fluid (or a very low fiber diet).

Though dehydration continues to be a much bigger problem related to water intake, it is important to know that you can get too much water. It is unlikely to happen in the backcountry if you are drinking and eating throughout the day, especially if you incorporate drink mixes when traveling in hot, humid environments. (See chapter 2 for information about hyponatremia, the condition that can occur with excessive fluid intake or over-hydration.)

Symptoms of Dehydration

Weakness	Constipation
Headache	Mental confusion
Fatigue	Increased heart rate
Lethargy	Decreased urine output

Risk Factors for Dehydration

Extreme heat, cold, humidity	Inadequate fluid intake
High altitude	Medications
High protein diet	Laxatives
High sodium diet	Diuretics (may include caffeine, varies according to use)
Vomiting, diarrhea	
Infection, fever	

HYPOTHERMIA AND FROSTBITE

Nutritional strategies to decrease your risk of developing cold injuries, such as hypothermia and frostbite, include avoiding alcohol and keeping yourself properly hydrated and fueled, so your body is able to generate heat as needed. Carbohydrate foods and drinks are easier to digest than fat or protein, and if you are having difficulty getting enough calories and fluid in cold weather conditions, combining the two may be a practical approach to better meet your needs. Once symptoms of hypothermia are present, warm sugar water is often recommended to assist with raising core temperature and providing energy to generate heat.

Risk Factors for Cold Injury According to the U.S. Military

Previous cold casualties (Clusters of cold casualties on prior days mean high risk for today.)
Use of tobacco/nicotine or alcohol in the last twenty-four hours
Skipping meals
Low activity
Fatigue/sleep deprivation
Little experience in cold weather
Dehydration
Minor illness (cold symptoms, sore throat, low-grade fever, nausea, vomiting), injuries, or wounds
Taking drugs (prescription, OTC, herbal, or dietary supplements)
Prior history of cold injury
Overly motivated soldiers (Overly motivated soldiers may not comply with cold casualty prevention measures.)

Hypothermia occurs when body temperature falls 1.8 to 3.6°F (1 to 2°C) below normal (98.6°F or 37°C). There are different stages, beginning with shivering, numbness, and inability to use hands properly due to restricted blood flow to the extremities; goose bumps; and quick, shallow breathing. As body temperature continues to drop, symptoms worsen and coordination becomes more difficult, confusion may begin, and complexion becomes pale. Symptoms progress until the body cannot move, and major organs shut down.

The major risk factors for hypothermia involve being unable to keep internal organs warm or to generate body heat. Low body fat, hypothyroidism, or decreased metabolism that occurs with age and certain medications also increase the risk of developing hypothermia. Additional risk factors are shown in the previous table.

HEAT INJURIES

Heat cramps, heat exhaustion, and heat stroke are potentially serious backcountry injuries that can occur in a variety of conditions. Hot and humid environments are the obvious places to suffer heat injuries due to excessive water and sodium losses through sweat. High levels of physical activity in the backcountry or particularly strenuous days may involve high sweat losses in any environment (high altitude, cold, or temperate). Excessive sun exposure can also lead to heat injuries in high-altitude environments.

The best nutritional strategy is similar to preventing cold injuries—stay well fueled and well hydrated. Additionally, if you are losing fluid through excessive sweating (remember, this may not be obvious in windy or dry climates where sweat evaporates quickly), you also need to make sure your foods include salt and perhaps plan to combine plain water with drink mixes that contain electrolytes. Drink mixes also contain carbohydrates and may help you drink more fluids than plain water.

CHAPTER 9 NUTRITION FOR EXTREME ENVIRONMENTS

After months of want and hunger, we suddenly found ourselves able to have meals fit for the gods, and with appetites the gods might have envied.
—Ernest Shackleton

The backcountry environment plays a major role in nutritional needs in the field. While the basics still apply (get enough food and fuel and you'll survive), there are some ways to prepare for travel in more extreme environments that are worth thinking about ahead of time. The three environmental challenges we'll review here are cold and hot environments and high altitude. There are similarities among these special environmental conditions, as well as a few important differences.

Military operations often involve exercise in high-altitude or hot or cold environmental conditions; therefore, the United States military has established the Committee on Military Nutrition Research and the Food and Nutrition Board that provides nutrition information for field personnel. The foundation of this chapter draws much information from the Institute of Medicine's *Nutritional Needs in Cold and in High-altitude Environments* and is supplemented by more recent published studies accessed through the Pub Med online research database.

HIGH-ALTITUDE ENVIRONMENT

High altitude refers to 5,000 feet (1,500 meters) above sea level or higher. Typically many of the negative symptoms associated with adjustment to higher altitudes (headaches, lightheadedness, and abnormal sleep patterns) occur for most people somewhere above 8,000 to 10,000 feet (2,438 to 3,000 meters), but there is a great deal of individual variability. The increased needs for both calories and fluid at higher altitudes, combined with the many challenges in meeting these needs, may contribute to these symptoms.

What is High Altitude?

High altitude = 5,000 to 11,500 feet (1,500 to 3,500 meters)
Very high altitude = 11,500 to 18,000 feet (3,500 to 5,500 meters)
Extreme altitude = 18,000 feet (5,500 meters) and above

Acclimatization to high altitude does occur for many individuals until extremely high altitude is reached. This process may take as little as a week, but the rate does vary among individuals. According to the International Society for Mountain Medicine, adjusting to high altitudes is mostly related to genetics and the rate of ascent. Age, sex, physical fitness, and previous altitude experience do not appear to be related to who gets acute mountain sickness (AMS) and who is able to acclimate more easily. There is no way to predict who will get sick at altitude. While there are no known nutritional links to developing altitude sickness, aiming for a nutritionally balanced diet, including plenty of fluids and foods that you enjoy, is important. Low blood sugar levels interfere with shivering, impairing your body's ability to generate heat, and in general, not getting enough food leads to the loss of muscle and fat.

Staying well fueled can also help you deal with other high-altitude challenges. High-altitude travel often involves a great deal of physical and psychological stress. Low blood sugar and even minor dehydration can affect your ability to think and act in these situations. In addition to the altitude itself, often there are extremely cold temperatures, wind, and dangerous terrain (snow, ice, crevasses, steep and exposed slopes) that require skill and strength to navigate.

Altitude Sickness

The American Heart Association recommends two days to reach 8,000 feet (2,438 meters) and one day for each additional 1,000 to 2,000 feet (305 to 610 meters).

Hypoxia: decreasing oxygen to meet needs

Altitude Sickness: symptoms include headaches, dizziness, lightheadedness, breathlessness, nausea, vomiting, loss of appetite, malaise, swelling of hands and feet.

Acute Mountain Sickness (AMS): symptoms include nausea, fatigue, headache, cough, loss of appetite, poor sleep, difficulty breathing at rest and while moving, fluid retention.

High-altitude Cerebral Edema (HACE): swelling and/or fluid accumulation in the brain; symptoms include changes in ability to think, confusion, staggering or stumbling as if intoxicated; fatal in hours or one to two days if not treated; person in this condition may not know he or she is ill; descend at least 1,600 to 3,300 feet (500 to 1,000 meters) to alleviate symptoms.

High-altitude Pulmonary Edema (HAPE): swelling and/or fluid accumulation in the lungs; symptoms include fast, shallow breathing (even at rest), extreme fatigue, coughing, chest tightening, gurgling or rattling breathing, blue or gray lips or fingernails, drowsiness; immediate descent and supplemental oxygen are critical.

FLUID REQUIREMENTS

At higher altitudes your heart and lungs need to work harder to deliver oxygen to your body's cells; also, the air is often very dry and cold. Heavy breathing just to walk in these conditions means you are losing more fluid through your lungs than when you are at sea level. In addition to the increases in both your respiratory and heart rate at high altitude, you must stay warm, as well as do whatever physical activity brought you to the backcountry. This means your body will require more fluid and more calories to get the job done.

In addition, you wear more clothing, possibly heavy boots, crampons, and mountaineering gear that adds weight and layers that contribute to sweat losses at altitude. You can lose as much water through sweat in an extremely cold environment as you do in hot and humid climates, and not realize it until you remove layers at the end of the day.

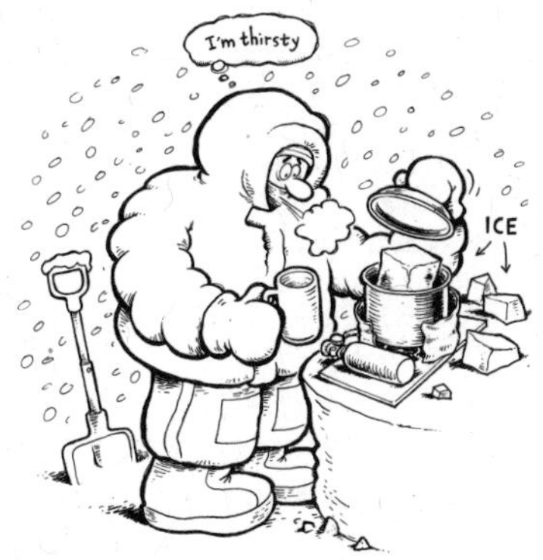

Another factor that affects your fluid requirements is excessive urination, technically referred to as altitude-induced diuresis. For those who experience diuresis (not everyone does), it is usually during the initial exposure to high altitude, and the severity of the losses varies from person to person. While some researchers attribute this side effect to the breakdown of both muscle and fat tissues, others believe diuresis may be a way to get rid of fluid in an attempt to prevent AMS. (See the Altitude Sickness table for more about AMS.) Either way, these water losses can contribute to dehydration.

The changes that occur while your body tries to adjust to high altitude, especially if you are physically active, mean that even if you drink enough fluid, it is possible that the fluids are *not* distributed the way they need to be within your body. It is also hard to imagine that you can have excess fluid in your brain or lungs yet be dehydrated, but it can happen. The best way to manage the more serious types of AMS, HACE, and HAPE (see the Altitude Sickness table) is to descend to a lower altitude.

One last factor related to fluid needs is that you require both food and water to provide fluid for metabolic reactions in your body. High altitude can decrease your appetite and ultimately your food intake. If you are not eating enough to meet your needs at high altitudes (and the higher you go the more likely this is), you need even more water. If you are working hard, your thirst indicators also may be suppressed (and, as discussed in the water chapter, you don't get thirsty until you are already dehydrated). Also, remember that dehydration is cumulative so you may hydrate adequately one day, then have a more active or cold day the next and not get enough fluid—and therefore begin the third day already inadequately hydrated.

► **During cold weather exercise (like skiing or mountaineering) keep snacks that can freeze in an inner pocket of your jacket where they will stay warm and be easy to access.**

According to U.S. Army research, constipation is a common complaint during any field exercise but is even more prevalent at high altitude. Decreased oxygen availability at altitude slows down the digestive system and the fluid losses discussed above take water from the colon, making it more difficult to move contents through the bowels. While responding to "nature's call" at high altitude may not be a pleasant experience, chronic constipation is not a great alternative. Aside from feeling miserable, this can also contribute to a decrease in food intake.

CALORIE NEEDS

Living and traveling at high altitudes requires more calories (energy) to move, as well as to fuel your basic metabolic functions, than living at sea level. The amount of additional calories you need varies according to the environmental temperature (extreme cold increases your needs even more), how much you are exercising, and your individual metabolic differences. A ballpark estimate for additional calories per day is roughly 300, just for basic bodily functions. Strenuous activity and extreme cold, however, can have much higher requirements. (Local mountaineers on an expedition to Denali forced themselves to eat 5,000 to 6,000 calories a day and still lost weight!)

did you know ?

The amount of caffeine in two cups of coffee (200 milligrams) may decrease blood flow to the heart during exercise at high altitude (study simulated 15,000 feet or 4,500 meters).

Unfortunately, appetite is often decreased or suppressed completely at higher altitudes, especially if you are experiencing symptoms of AMS. The higher you go, the more you are likely to suffer a decrease in appetite. Eating smaller, more frequent meals and snacks is key to keeping up with your calorie needs. It is important to remember here that losing weight on an expedition is not a good thing. If you are not meeting your basic calorie needs, you will lose both fat (needed to stay warm) and muscle (needed to move, work, and live). At altitudes around 16,500 feet (5,000 meters) it is difficult to maintain body weight even if you are eating and drinking consistently.

> **did you know ?**
>
> Your food intake may be reduced by 10 to 50 percent at very high altitude (varies among individuals and rate of ascent).

The most important factor for high-altitude menus is palatability. Choose foods you love at home, and even though they may not taste the same at high altitude, you probably will continue to find these foods palatable. When planning your food, think about things like limited water to make meals (especially if you must melt snow for both drinking and eating), limited fuel to cook, and the fact that even basic camp chores usually will require more physical and mental energy than at lower altitudes. Pack snacks that are easy to eat, carry, and that taste good to you. Salty and spicy foods may be more appealing, unless the altitude makes you feel nauseous, in which case you may want more bland foods.

As mentioned before, keeping blood sugar levels steady is important in order to think clearly, make good decisions, fuel your body (brain and muscles), and keep the crabby moods to a minimum, which contributes to good EB (expedition behavior). It is extremely important to remember that eating small, frequent meals and snacks can help with energy and blood sugar levels. Keep easy-to-eat foods that you enjoy in pockets that are easy to access and readily available fluids where they will not freeze. You may need to create a schedule for eating and drinking throughout the day if you experience a decrease in appetite and thirst.

CARBOHYDRATES AND FAT

In addition to enough calories and water, getting enough carbohydrate at high altitude is important. Carbohydrate is the primary fuel, both at rest and during exercise at high altitude. It takes less oxygen to burn carbohydrate than fat or protein. This doesn't mean fat and protein aren't important. As the fat chapter points out, one of the roles of fat in food is to make it taste good. Food that tastes good can help you keep up with your nutrition needs at altitude. A variety of foods that contain pro-

► **On cold days fill a water bottle with hot tea and some honey to provide a nice, warm drink with some carbohydrate for energy.**

tein, fat, and carbohydrates will help you meet your nutritional needs and make eating more interesting. Also, higher energy needs at altitude means that excluding fat from your diet may make it difficult or impossible to meet your calorie needs.

While the idea persists that people venturing into high-altitude environments prefer high carbohydrate to high fat foods, and that we may not be able to properly digest high-fat foods at these altitudes, current research does not consistently support either of these ideas. There is a great deal of individual variability in both preferences for foods and tolerance of them. While fat metabolism does require more oxygen than carbohydrate, it is not clear that malabsorption is related to difficulty getting enough calories at altitude, especially at the altitudes most commonly accessed by skiers and hikers. Extremely high altitudes (above 18,000 feet or 5,500 meters) may be a different story.

There are some high carbohydrate foods that are very popular among mountaineers and climbers, but many of these foods are low in calories so a diet consisting largely of these foods would not supply enough calories for living and exercising at high altitudes. One example is ramen noodles that provide fluid and salt in addition to the carbohydrates, are quick and easy to prepare, and appeal to many high-altitude adventurers. However, a whole package contains only about 300 calories, more of a snack than a meal for a trip with high calorie needs. One AT hiker included ramen on his "worst foods" list, claiming "they had no umph . . . you get what you pay for." Of course, you can use ramen as a base for a meal, adding cheese for fat and protein, maybe some dried veggies, and some crackers or bread along with it for more substance.

did you know ?

A high carbohydrate diet before and during initial exposure to high altitude may improve your mood and performance.

As in all backcountry situations, carbohydrates are important to fuel your muscles and your brain. At altitude they are also most easily and efficiently converted to fuel with the limited oxygen available. Even the easy-to-prepare carbohydrate foods that don't provide a lot of calories can make a great snack or base for a meal at altitude. It comes back to making sure you are eating and drinking consistently at altitude, even when you don't feel like it.

PROTEIN

While some studies have shown losses of lean body mass at high altitudes, suggesting a higher need for protein, other research shows a loss of both lean and fat mass. The general thinking at this point is that if you get enough calories at altitude from a mixed diet, there is no evidence to support a greater need for protein. In fact, eating more protein requires additional water to process the metabolic byproducts of protein breakdown. Since fluid requirements are already increased at altitude, and water sources are often limited in alpine environments, a high protein intake is probably not the best nutritional choice.

VITAMINS AND MINERALS

The need for supplemental vitamins for high-altitude backcountry travel is not clear at this point. Because appetite is decreased and getting enough calories is challenging at altitude, if you are planning an extended high-altitude expedition (more than three to four weeks) a multivitamin and mineral supplement may be a good insurance policy. This could ensure that you are getting iron, zinc, some of the B vitamins your body doesn't store, and a basic assortment of antioxidants (A, C, E, selenium), all of which are important for exercise at altitude.

Making sure your iron stores are normal is also a good idea prior to a trek to high altitude, especially for women, since there is an increased need for red blood cells at high altitude. Iron is part of hemoglobin, the major oxygen transporter in red blood cells. There is a temporary increase in iron absorption at high altitude to satisfy this increased need. (See chapter 6 for backcountry food sources of iron.)

► **Sunflower seeds are an excellent source of vitamin E. Sunflower seed butter is a great alternative to peanut butter. This yummy spread is also a good source of B vitamins, magnesium, iron, zinc and fiber.**

There have been studies of high-altitude mountaineers that show an increase in zinc losses in the urine at very high altitude (27,726 feet or 8,451 meters). Like iron, there is also an increase in the intestinal absorption of zinc that may compensate for this loss, but it is not known if this mechanism is enough to offset the zinc losses.

There is some research to support possible benefits of a supplemental mixture of antioxidant vitamins and minerals to reduce oxidative stress that can occur at high altitude. Oxidative stress occurs when too many free radicals and other reactive compounds are formed for the body to process with its antioxidant systems. In addition to the limited amount of oxygen getting to tissues at altitude, there is exposure to UV light, extreme cold, and psychological stress that contribute to the formation of these potentially damaging compounds (see chapter 6 for more information about antioxidants).

Not all studies have shown antioxidant supplements to be effective in decreasing oxidative stress, and it isn't clear that oxidative stress is always a bad thing (it may be part of your body's adjustment to high altitude). The jury is still out about whether or not to recommend supplements to possibly prevent the long-term damage to cells caused by oxidative stress. What you eat prior to going to high altitude does seem to play a role in whether or not supplements help. In at least one study, the only benefits of antioxidant supplementation appeared to be among some of the individuals with low antioxidant status (that reflects a poor diet) prior to the study.

There is some interesting research regarding vitamin E supplementation well above the RDA (400 milligrams per day). Vitamin E may decrease lipid peroxidation, one of the potentially damaging processes spurred by high altitude that can be detrimental to health and athletic performance.

did you know?

Absorbing fats, carbohydrates, and protein is not a common problem at elevations frequently reached by recreational skiers and backpackers.

Early studies related to vitamin C showed decreased tissue concentrations of vitamin C in simulated high-altitude environments (with guinea pigs) and increased urinary excretion

Specific Food Notes for High Altitude

When planning your high-altitude menu there are a few things to remember:

Perishability—consider how the food will get from your kitchen to the mountains when choosing foods for a cold, high-altitude environment. It is tempting to include foods that will not perish in a colder climate, but if perishable food will not be kept refrigerated prior to arriving at your high-altitude camp where it is cold enough to prevent bacteria from growing, then leave it at home.

Pre-field meals—if you are traveling to a developing country, be careful not to eat raw salads or fruit that cannot be peeled, local street foods, ice cream, etc., and do not drink untreated water or drinks with ice prior to entering the field. These are all high-risk foods for pathogens that can make you sick. Remember also that symptoms of food-borne illness may not occur until days after you have eaten or drunk the offensive food or drink. (See chapter 8 for more about food-borne illness in the backcountry.)

Hydration packs—these are a convenient way to carry water and help you drink more often in the backcountry, but at high altitudes and in cold environments it is difficult to keep the tubes from freezing (even with insulated covering). Ideally you can experiment ahead of time with hydration systems in a cold environment (skiing or winter camping, etc.), but if not, stick to water bottles that can be kept close to your body to keep from freezing. (Even with an acceptable hydration pack, an extra water bottle is good for drink mix or tea and provides a backup if the hydration pack is damaged.)

Drink mixes—these are a great way to add carbohydrate and sodium, and to make water taste better if you boil it or use iodine tablets for purification. Remember to wait a full thirty minutes after treating water with iodine, chlorine, or halogen before adding the powdered mix, which can interfere with the chemical reaction that kills the pathogen.

of vitamin C in humans. Currently, there isn't enough research to say that these changes happen consistently at altitude or what amounts of vitamin C may be needed to offset these losses. Vitamin C does play a role in regenerating vitamin E in the body, making it available to do more free radical scavenging. This may be part of the reason that mixtures of antioxidants seem to provide more protection at altitude than single high-dose antioxidants. In the meantime, including drink mixes fortified with vitamin C in your high-altitude rations is a way to supplement this vitamin while also tending to your fluid needs.

Getting enough of the water-soluble B vitamins involved in energy production (thiamin, niacin, riboflavin, pantothenic acid) is also important at high altitude. Unless you are spending more than three to four weeks at high altitude, supplementation is probably not necessary if you eat a variety of foods and focus on getting enough fuel.

COLD ENVIRONMENTS

There are many similarities between high altitude and cold environments, since they often occur together. This section will emphasize the differences between the two and refer to previous sections of this book for several points.

FLUID REQUIREMENTS

Fluid requirements increase in cold environments for several reasons. Merely breathing in cold temperatures increases water needs because cold air contains less moisture than warmer air, especially at higher altitudes. This means more fluid has to leave the lungs to humidify the cold, dry air and then warm it to body temperature. In the cold you may need an additional liter of fluid a day, and this does not include what you may need for exercise.

Many people experience cold-induced diuresis (similar to the high-altitude-induced diuresis), an increase in fluid losses via excessive urination. Again, this varies among individuals regarding the amount of fluid lost, and it may or may not occur. Sometimes it is an immediate reaction upon entering the cold and then, once your body has adjusted to the temperature, things return to normal.

Travel in cold environments often involves heavy gear and bulky clothing, increasing sweat losses that you may not be aware of until you undress at the end of the day. Sweat losses in the cold can be the same as in hot, humid environments.

CALORIE NEEDS

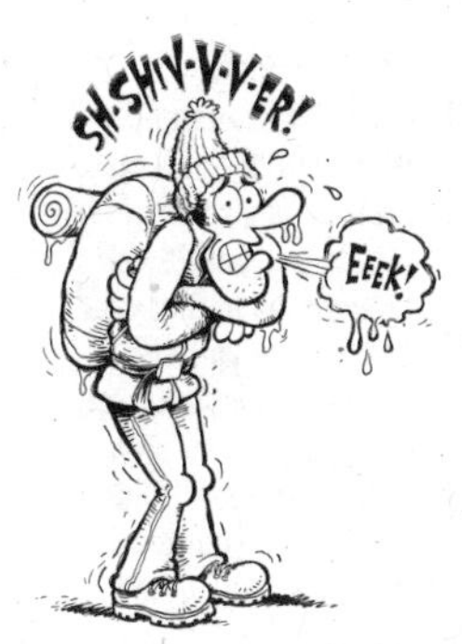

Another aspect of body temperature regulation (thermoregulation) that contributes to the increased calorie (energy) needs in the cold is shivering. Shivering is your body's way of producing heat and may increase energy needs more than twofold. Low blood sugar levels, from not getting enough fuel throughout the day, can impair shivering and increase your risk of hypothermia (see chapter 8 for more about cold injuries). The U.S. military has determined energy expenditure in the cold is between 3,400 and 4,300 calories per day, depending upon the degree of exposure. The military RDA for energy in cold environments is 4,500 calories per day. The NOLS winter rations are in line with this recommendation as well.

Cold environments do not generally have the same effect on appetite as high altitude. Appetite is often increased in the cold, and maintaining body weight is less difficult if adequate calories are available and easy to prepare, including appropriate shelter for food preparation. Unfortunately, cold and high-altitude environments are often combined, and the combination of decreased appetite (even with hunger there is often a decreased desire to eat) with increased caloric needs means unwanted weight loss that can make it difficult for your body to adjust to the cold. Remember that losing weight means losing fat and muscle, and you need both on a cold-weather expedition.

In general, while the number of calories needed increases dramatically in cold environments (especially when exercising or working in the cold), the amount of carbohydrate, protein and fat needed does not vary significantly from general recommendations for physically active individuals in more temperate climates. Although many cite the high fat content of indigenous Arctic populations as an indication that this diet is somehow su-

did you know ?

Low blood sugar in cold environments suppresses shivering, making it difficult for your body to stay warm.

► **Hard candies (Jolly Ranchers and Werther's butterscotch) are an easy, convenient way to get simple carbohydrates to fuel your brain when you don't have an appetite or you need to push on without stopping for food (just brush your teeth well when you get to camp).**

perior for survival in the cold, research doesn't support this idea. The choice of foods is often limited in extremely cold, remote environments like the Arctic, and is most likely the reason for dietary choices. Again, a higher fat diet than is generally recommended in the front-country (approximately 35 percent of daily calories from fat) is appropriate and may even be needed to get enough calories, but a mixed diet is still the goal.

CARBOHYDRATES AND FAT

Carbohydrates are still important for energy, but there is generally a better tolerance for fat in the cold compared to high altitude. Even if the cold climate is not at high altitude, carbohydrate is more readily converted to energy than fat or protein. Fat will help you meet your increased energy requirements in the cold, since fat metabolism yields nine calories per gram versus four calories per gram for carbohydrate and protein. A sudden change to a high fat diet, however, may cause gastrointestinal distress and other side effects. If you know you are going to a cold environment where you will benefit from a higher fat diet, particularly if you have a sensitive digestive system, it may be a good idea to increase your fat intake gradually prior to your trip. This can help your body to adjust to a higher fat diet to meet your need for more calories.

As mentioned above, low blood sugar can negatively affect your ability to generate body heat via shivering. Eating carbohydrates throughout the day at meals and snacks will help you keep your muscles fueled and your liver glycogen stores full to feed your brain.

PROTEIN

Although fat is often touted as the nutrient of choice to keep warm in cold environments, protein metabolism generates more body heat than either carbohydrate or fat, making adequate protein important for warmth. In many backcountry staples (cheese, nuts, seeds, or jerky), protein and fat often occur together; therefore, the fact that the protein is actually providing more warmth may not be obvious. At least one study has shown an increase in body warmth for five to six hours following a high protein meal. A protein snack prior to sleep may provide additional warmth in the cold from the thermal effect of protein metabolism. This does not mean a high-protein diet is appropriate for cold environments, however. Keep in mind that you need readily available energy from carbohydrates, and with increased water needs in the cold, you don't want a high protein diet that requires even more water.

The U.S. military recommendation for protein in the cold is 100 grams per 4,650 calories. Essentially, the amount of protein required is the same as in temperate climes, but the overall percentage of total calories from protein is lower (9 percent in cold climate versus 12.5 percent in temperate climates).

VITAMINS AND MINERALS

There is little research to support the need for vitamins and minerals above the RDA to help your body adapt to the cold. One study published in 1949 proposed that vitamin C may play a role in maintaining body core and surface temperatures, but the study has never been confirmed. Adequate intakes of the B vitamins involved in energy metabolism is once again important (thiamin, niacin, riboflavin, pantothenic acid) and chronic deficiencies of trace elements such as zinc, iron, and copper may lead to problems with thermoregulation. But, once again, if you get enough calories from a mixed diet, you will probably get enough of these nutrients. If you are planning an expedition that will last more than a month in an extreme environment, a multivitamin and mineral supplement should be enough to prevent a micronutrient deficiency.

HOT ENVIRONMENTS

Hot environments are more nutritionally challenging than temperate climates; this is because increased water needs and a decreased appetite can make getting enough calories difficult.

FLUID REQUIREMENTS

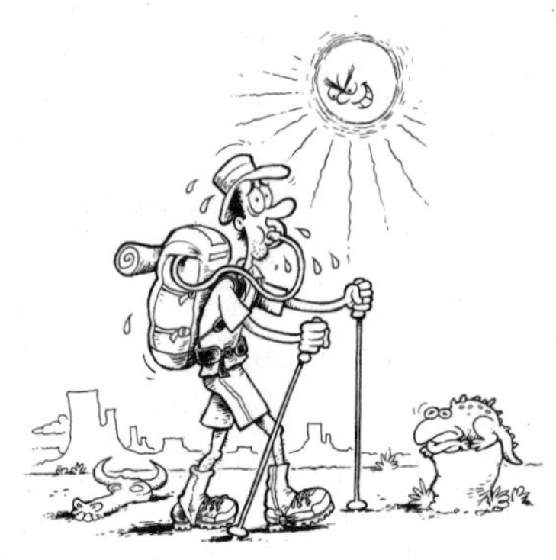

The most important, and probably the most obvious, nutritional requirement that changes in hot environments is fluid intake. Heavy sweat losses occur during prolonged exercise in the heat and are intensified in the backcountry by strenuous exercise like carrying a heavy pack or climbing gear. Although this is obvious in hot, humid situations when sweat is literally dripping down your back, it may be less obvious in dry heat and wind that quickly evaporate sweat. This is common in hot, high-altitude environments where it is dry and often windy.

In the heat, up to 3 liters of fluid may be lost per hour through sweat. This is approximately 50 milliliters per minute, and only 20 to 30 milliliters of fluid per minute may be absorbed from the intestines. This means you cannot absorb fluid fast enough to replace the fluid you lose exercising in hot environments. So, you must drink before, during, and after physical activity in the heat to keep up with your fluid needs. It is also best to drink small amounts of fluid throughout the day rather than large amounts every once in a while.

Water is the number one nutritional concern to prepare for a backcountry trip into a hot environment. You can refer to chapter 2 for detailed information about the importance of water and electrolytes, how much you need, and which foods (and beverages) provide electrolytes. Chapter 2 also discusses hyponatremia, the situation that arises with excessive salt losses combined with fluid overload or dehydration. It all comes back to balance. We need enough water, and dehydration is certainly the more common challenge in the backcountry, but excessive intake of plain water

did you know ?

Cold fluids cool your body's core temperature and may make you drink more in the heat.

combined with heavy sweating can lead to low blood-sodium levels, a potentially life-threatening condition.

CALORIE NEEDS

Many people experience a decrease in appetite when exercising in hot weather. As your body's core temperature rises, your appetite decreases. This means you may need to schedule meals and snacks as you would in high-altitude environments, since you cannot rely on feeling hungry. Ideally, you would have access to fresh foods with a higher water content, such as fresh fruit, salads, and grilled fish, which are more appealing in hot weather. The reality is, unless you are venturing into tropical areas with fruit trees and a body of water to provide fish nearby, you probably won't have this luxury. So eating small amounts of whatever food you can make yourself eat throughout the day, along with lots of fluid, can help. Drink mixes or packets of lemon flavoring added to water can help you drink more fluid. It is easy to get bored with drinking plain water when your needs are so high (often 5 to 6 liters or more a day). Drink mixes can also add carbohydrate (usually some kind of sugar) and sodium (salt and chloride) to help with glycogen stores and electrolyte balance. Be aware that not all sports drinks contain enough sodium for long days of sweating. In the backcountry when you also have access to salty foods, this may not be a problem. However, you can lose more than 1,000 milligrams of sodium per hour in sweat (½ teaspoon of salt contains 1,200 milligrams of sodium). While there are no hard and fast recommendations for replacing sodium, if you are sweating a lot (if it is windy, you may not realize how much you are sweating), make sure you are getting sodium in foods and drinks throughout the day. This will help you stimulate your thirst sensors and retain water.

Using salt tablets in hot environments to replace losses in sweat is usually not necessary if you eat enough food throughout the day. Many common backcountry foods are packaged or canned and contain high amounts of

> ► **In warm weather climates be careful with trail mix that includes chocolate chips—you may end up with a big gooey mess.**

Common Backcountry Foods High in Sodium (Salt)

Ramen noodles
Soup mixes
Dehydrated, packaged meals
Salted nuts and seeds
Pretzels, crackers
Jerky (made from beef, turkey, or fish)
Canned tuna, chicken, seafood, meat

sodium so you will be getting a good amount of salt from meals and snacks. (Salt tablets typically contain 200 to 350 milligrams of sodium and an ounce of cheese has over 400 milligrams.)

If your appetite is suppressed or you are recovering from an illness that caused you to eat less than usual, you may want to add some salt to your water or keep salt tablets handy. Another strategy if you are concerned about getting enough salt is to include a cup of broth or bouillon with an afternoon snack or at the end of the day, and add extra salt (or soy sauce or other salty condiments) to your evening meal. This is especially helpful if your backcountry foods are less packaged or processed with less salt.

SPECIFIC NUTRIENTS

The recommendations for both macro- and micronutrients in hot environments do not differ significantly from more temperate climates. The situation is similar to both the high-altitude and cold environments in that if you get enough calories from a mixed diet, you are most likely getting plenty of the carbohydrate, fat, protein, vitamins, and minerals that you need for a hot environment.

FINAL THOUGHTS FOR THE FIELD

Traveling in extreme backcountry environments presents many nutritional challenges. Your need for fluid is higher in all three situations described in this chapter, but often when your calorie needs are high, your appetite is low. The idea that you need to schedule food and drink, when you are not hungry or thirsty, is counter intuitive and flies in the face of much nutritional advice you are given in the frontcountry.

While getting enough of the various nutrients needed to adapt to these environments is important, in many ways the extreme climates force us back to survival mode. While the premise of this book is to take you beyond survival, in the case of extreme environments, I fully embrace the idea of eating what you can, and will, as your first goal. My husband remembers planning his expedition menu for Denali based on the high-carbohydrate recommendations for high altitude, and then being the envy of other groups as he made cheese quesadillas at 16,000 feet. As with so many adventures in life, the theory is good to know, but practice is where you learn what works best for you.

CHAPTER 10

NUTRITION FOR TEENS

Children have more need of models than of critics.
—Carolyn Coats, author of children's books

The backcountry experience is an incredible educational opportunity for children and teens. During the past couple of decades the number of outdoor programs has risen dramatically and many, like NOLS, offer extended trips in the field with a variety of options for physical activity. Because children and adolescents are growing and developing, they have needs beyond the normal recommendations for endurance activities. Because the focus of this book is nutritional considerations for extended backcountry travel, this section will focus on adolescents, rather than children, given the very small number of preadolescents likely to participate in long backcountry trips. For ease in writing (and reading), hereafter in this chapter I will refer to this population as teens.

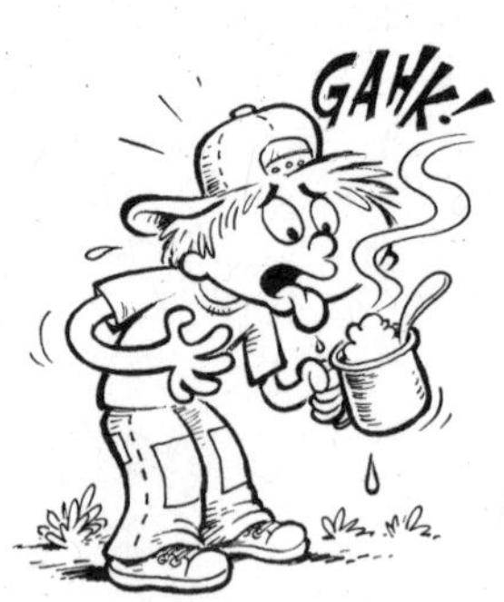

As with adults traveling into the backcountry, if teens begin the trip well nourished, it is unlikely any nutrient deficiencies will develop. Getting enough calories from a variety of foods is, once again, the best way to ensure that young backcountry adventurers will get enough of the various nutrients. This may be easier in theory than in practice with teens in the field, particularly if they are picky eaters. While adults seem willing and able to adjust their nutrition for long-term health benefits, this isn't typical for kids and teens. If, however, teens are educated about the specific short-term benefits of good backcountry nutrition and how to achieve these goals, they are much more likely to engage in planning and eating well in the field. In addition to emphasizing food as fuel it may help to clearly establish what eating well will do for a teen traveler now, today, in the present, versus some future health risk.

> **► Make your own backcountry ketchup with tomato powder, sugar, and vinegar (vinegar is a great addition to your spice kit). Combining a familiar flavor like this can help young picky eaters in the backcountry enjoy new foods.**

What Eating Well in the Field Can Do for You

Give you more energy throughout the day for exercise and maintaining camp
Boost your immune system to fight illness and stay healthy
Provide the nutrients needed to build muscle (and burn fat)
Be a good incentive to learn to cook
Provide good social time preparing and sharing group meals

Nutritional Concerns Related to Teens in the Backcountry

Unwilling to try new foods, particularly some of the foods needed for key nutrients like protein, iron, and calcium (meal mixes that contain beans and legumes, powdered milk, alternative nut butters, etc.)
Unaware of symptoms related to dehydration and low blood sugar
May not eat enough due to body image concerns, not realizing the amount of calories they need to support their backcountry activities (especially young girls)
Accustomed to eating only at prescribed times and have trouble with the idea that backcountry travelers need to fuel regularly throughout the day
May not be assertive enough to express needs for food and fluid, perhaps relying on adults in the group to initiate such things as rest and fuel stops and eating times
May not know how to cook, thus cook foods improperly

FLUID REQUIREMENTS

The fluid requirements for teens do not differ significantly from adults, a baseline of 3 to 4 liters per day, including a combination of plain water and other backcountry beverages. The challenge here may be making fluids more palatable since teens are likely to be less experienced with the need to drink before they are thirsty. Drink mixes and a pleasing beverage temperature (cold water for hot climates and warm drinks for cold climates) may help increase fluid consumption for teens (and adults).

CALORIE NEEDS

There are differences in the timing of developmental changes between boys and girls. By the time girls reach adolescence they may have already peaked in terms of growth, since they typically experience a growth spurt between ages ten and eleven, peaking at age twelve. For boys the spurt is often later, say twelve to thirteen, peaking at age fourteen. Even though both boys and girls may continue to grow throughout the teenage years, their need for additional calories is more dependent upon their physical activity than their needs for growth.

The difference between basic calorie needs (to estimate Resting Energy Expenditure see the following table) for a girl or boy ages ten to seventeen versus eighteen to twenty-nine is only about 115 calories more for the younger age group. Physical activity, on the other hand, can increase calorie needs in the backcountry by 1,000 to 3,000 depending on the environmental conditions and the activity. (See chapter 1 or appendix D for more information about how to estimate calorie needs for a day in the backcountry.)

> ▶ **Teens may be more interested in backcountry nutrition when they know what it can do for them on a daily basis (they are less likely to be motivated by things like preventing heart disease when they are older).**

This information is important for the young backcountry traveler, especially if he or she has a history of restricting calories in the frontcountry for weight management purposes. The restriction could

Estimation of the Daily Resting Energy Expenditure (REE)

Age (years)	*Equation*
Males	
10–17	(17.5 × body weight*) + 651
18–29	(15.3 × body weight) + 679
30–60	(11.6 × body weight) + 879
Females	
10–17	(12.2 × body weight*) + 746
18–29	(14.7 × body weight) + 496
30–60	(8.7 × body weight) + 829

REE does not include calories needed for physical activity—this is the baseline of calories used for basic functions.

*Weight in kilograms (kg) (kg = pounds divided by 2.2; e.g., 150 lbs. ÷ 2.2 = 68 kg)

be for health, body image, or sports performance reasons, and may or may not be identified as a problem. Teens must know that this behavior related to food is not acceptable in the backcountry and may have serious consequences. Remember, getting enough fluid and calories are the top nutritional priorities in the backcountry for both survival and enjoyment. Encouraging younger members of the group to do some calculations to estimate the calories they will need in the backcountry, and then looking at some examples of what that amount of calories looks like in terms of food, can be very enlightening.

Once you know roughly how many calories you need in the backcountry and the amount of food you need to eat to get that many calories, it is clear that eating throughout the day is a logical way to meet your nutritional needs. This may be another challenge for teens since they may think the fact that schools don't acknowledge the need for snacking during the day once students are out of elementary school (a major problem in my view) means they aren't supposed to need snacks. The implication is that as we get older, we don't need snacks. Unfortunately this isn't necessarily true in the frontcountry, and it is definitely not true during backcountry days that include several hours of exercise. Fueling throughout the day is critical to keep blood sugar levels steady, which keeps energy levels high and the brain thinking clearly.

Once again, the emphasis on food as fuel for activity needs to be clear. It is equally important to make sure young backcountry travelers are aware of the symptoms of both dehydration and low blood sugar (refer to water and carbohydrate sections for lists of symptoms). It should be plainly stated that all group members, regardless of age or experience, must care for their nutritional needs for water and food. Some younger group members may feel shy about stopping even if they know they need to refuel or hydrate. Again, let them know that self-care contributes to the success and enjoyment of the whole group. Getting grumpy or (worse) sick because of poor nutritional habits is much more of an inconvenience to the expedition than a five to ten minute rest stop to eat and drink.

PROTEIN

While many nutrition experts believe young athletes need more protein than nonathletes do to provide for growth and increased physical activity, there is no specific research to support this idea. Still, the fact that protein is needed to build new tissues, above and beyond that required for exercise, suggests it is a good idea for kids and teens to aim for the upper end of protein recommendations.

Protein Recommendations for Youths

.6 to .9 grams of protein per pound (1.3 to 2 grams per kilogram) per day for competitive athletes, growing teenage athletes, and adults restricting calories or building muscle mass

.45 to .41 grams of protein per pound (1 to .9 grams per kilogram) for nonathletes ages seven to eighteen

OTHER NUTRIENTS

The need for carbohydrates and fat are not significantly different during the teen years in general. As with adults venturing into the backcountry, it is important that teens understand the facts about carbohydrates as fuel for exercise and are not consciously or subconsciously avoiding or limiting carbohydrates. This is also true regarding fat, especially if there is a reluctance to eat high fat foods such as nuts, seeds, nut butters (peanut butter, almond butter, etc.), and cheese. These foods are often major sources of protein, calories and a wide array of important vitamins, minerals, and plant compounds (phytonutrients) in the backcountry.

Iron is important for making new red blood cells to deliver oxygen to working muscles and is related to both exercise performance and immune system function. There is some research that suggests iron supplementation may be beneficial to athletic young children and teens, but at this point that decision needs to be made by a pediatrician or dietitian on an individual basis. There is not enough evidence to make a blanket recommendation about iron supplements in the backcountry. The fact that these supplements can cause other problems in the backcountry—i.e., constipation and possibly contribute to oxidative stress—suggests iron supplements need to be carefully considered. Young girls that have begun to menstruate should check their iron stores prior to going into the field, since they will have higher needs for iron between growth and monthly losses.

Roughly 25 to 30 percent of total bone mass is stored during the adolescent years, so getting enough calcium and vitamin D is also important, though this is more of a long-term consideration than a short-term backcountry need. The need for other vitamins and minerals is similar to adults in that if teens get enough calories from a variety of foods, their higher needs in the backcountry will be met.

FINAL THOUGHTS FOR THE FIELD

The backcountry can be an incredible classroom for teens and, as with adults, good nutrition can increase the enjoyment of the backcountry experience. If teens have little or no experience preparing and cooking food prior to going into the field, or are not familiar with the foods included in the field rations, it may help to suggest some easy-to-prepare and familiar foods at the beginning of the trip. Macaroni and cheese, pasta, and chili are some ideas, but including teens in meal planning is an important part of the process.

Lastly, don't underestimate the importance of being a good role model. In many cases, what you do in the backcountry will be more important than what you say. In my experience, telling kids and teens what to eat for good health does not work as well as showing them how to do it by eating well in their presence.

CHAPTER 11

SPECIAL DIETS

Nothing is particularly hard if you divide it into small steps.
—Henry Ford

The various links between what we eat and our health are not new; "you are what you eat" has been a common adage for decades. However, the increased number of overweight and obesity cases—in combination with increases in many chronic diseases like heart disease, diabetes, and cancer—has inspired more people than ever to take a closer look at what they eat. Another factor contributing to special diets is that more people are being proactive about their health, seeking ways to prevent illness in addition to treating symptoms. There are also environmental concerns, spiritual beliefs, and just plain old food preferences that lead some to exclude certain foods from their diets.

There also has been an increased awareness of food-related intolerances, sensitivities, allergies, and other conditions. Celiac disease, for example, is now estimated to affect 1 in 133 people in the U.S., though many still go undiagnosed. Lactose intolerance, when the body doesn't make enough of the enzyme needed to break down the lactose sugar in dairy foods, is also common among adults.

This section will address a few common special dietary concerns, some that are based on medical or health issues and others related more to personal preferences. It is important to remember that, in the backcountry, getting enough fluid and enough calories from a variety of foods is the key to optimal

> ▶ **Vegetarian chili mixes often contain textured soy protein (also called textured vegetable protein, or TVP) that can be difficult to digest, especially if you are a little dehydrated. Try soaking the mix in the cook water for a while prior to cooking or allow cooked chili to sit covered for an extra five to ten minutes after cooking (to save fuel).**

nutrition to support your athletic performance, physical health, and emotional well-being. The more flexible you are with your eating habits, the easier it is going to be for you (and your expedition mates) to successfully fuel yourself. It is possible to get all of the nutrients you need with any of the special diets included in this section, but some require more careful planning, creativity, and a willingness to expand your food choices than when you are at home.

Backcountry nutrition may differ dramatically from everyday recommendations in that there are many factors to balance when designing your menu. While health and nutritional concerns are important (hence the need for a book like this!), there are other things that must be considered, such as pack weight, water and fuel needed to prepare and clean up after meals, and perishability (refer to chapter 1 for a full list). There are also nutrients, such as sodium, that are needed in larger amounts when backcountry travel involves major losses of sodium through sweat. Often calorie, carbohydrate, and protein needs are much higher for the active backcountry adventurer than for the average person. If you have a specific medical issue that requires a modified diet, the best thing to do is to consult with a Registered Dietitian (RD) who has experience with sports nutrition and knowledge about backcountry needs. Some of the recommendations you may have been given to manage your condition may need to be adjusted for the backcountry.

VEGETARIAN DIETS

Vegetarian diets were once associated with counterculture, hippies, and health nuts or thought to be inspired by environmental, spiritual, or health reasons. Mainstream culture, including the medical and nutrition communities, was skeptical about the viability of a vegetarian eating style to provide all of the necessary nutrients for good health. In fact, the first time that the Dietary Guidelines for Americans acknowledged that some vegetarian diets are consistent with excellent health was not until 1995. There is still skepticism regarding the stricter versions of vegetarian diets, such as vegans and fruitarians, mainly because any severely restrictive diet makes it difficult to get everything you need nutritionally. However, vegetarianism is more widely accepted, and it is now common to see entrees in restaurants and many choices in the frozen food aisle to accommodate vegetarians or those who just wish to eat more plant foods.

Variations of Vegetarian Diets

Fruitarian—eats only raw or dried fruits, seeds, and nuts
Lacto vegetarian—eats dairy products, vegetables, grains, legumes, fruits, and nuts
Ovo vegetarian—eats eggs, vegetables, grains, legumes, fruits, and nuts
Pesco vegetarian—eats seafood, vegetables, grains, legumes, fruits, and nuts
Vegan (or strict vegetarian)—eats only food from plant sources: vegetables, grains, legumes, fruits, seeds, and nuts

Many common backcountry foods fit into some type of vegetarian diet. The NOLS standard rations basically provide a modified vegetarian diet. The cheese, powdered milk, and egg (the egg is used for backcountry baking) classify this variation as a lacto-ovo vegetarian diet (includes dairy and eggs). Some winter and semester courses include packaged or canned fish or poultry, and students and instructors may opt to bring jerky or canned meats to supplement the standard rations.

Some of the hikers who responded to an Appalachian Trail nutrition survey (see appendix G) found it difficult to find vegetarian options in many of the towns along the trail. While this may have changed somewhat during the past several years (the survey was conducted in 2000), with obesity on the rise and more people paying attention to their diets, this is a consideration when you are resupplying on a long trip. You may need to arrange for foods to be sent or delivered to various places along the way or be creative in small towns that may not have a lot of vegetarian options. My first thought, however, when reading the surveys was that you may not find a variety of creative "vegetarian-specific" packaged meals but you can almost always find a market or grocery store with bread and peanut butter.

► Add a pinch of cayenne pepper or Mexican spice mix to powdered hummus to enhance the taste (cayenne pepper is also good for your immune system). Pack the dry hummus (with or without added spice) with your trail foods and add water when you stop for food.

PROTEIN

Although protein is still often mentioned as the nutrient likely to be deficient in a vegetarian diet, the truth is there are many plant sources of protein and getting enough, even for the very active backcountry traveler, is not difficult with a vegetarian diet. The protein section discusses the issue of complete versus incomplete proteins, but basically, animal foods contain protein that has all of the amino acids (in adequate amounts) that our bodies cannot make and therefore must get from food. Plant proteins are considered incomplete proteins, with the exception of soybeans and some foods made from soybeans (tofu, tempeh, textured soy protein, etc.). This just means you need a variety of plant proteins that combine to provide enough of the essential amino acids.

At one time, people thought that complementary proteins from different plant foods needed to be combined at one time to get the benefits of a complete protein. This has long since been debunked, yet I am still asked about combining foods to make complete proteins. It just happens that there are many logical and delicious combinations that do combine to make a complete protein such as rice and beans or whole wheat bread and peanut butter (see the Complementary Protein Combinations table). The best approach is to eat a varied diet. If you choose not to eat dairy or eggs (already complete proteins that increase the protein value of any plant foods consumed along with them), then make sure beans, lentils, nuts, seeds, and grains are part of your daily fare.

Complementary Protein Combinations

Grains and legumes

- Rice and beans
- Wheat bread and peanut butter
- Corn tortillas and refried beans
- Hummus (chick peas and sesame seed paste)

Milk and grains or legumes

- Pasta and milk or cheese
- Cereal with milk
- Macaroni and cheese
- Cheese and refried beans

The protein chapter in section I includes a table with the amount of protein in some common backcountry foods, and appendix C lists the various foods in the standard NOLS rations, including the amount of protein. From these lists you can see that compared to animal foods, plant sources of protein do have less per serving. Using the protein recommendations for endurance athletes (slightly higher than those used for the average couch potato) to estimate your daily protein needs, multiply your weight in pounds by both .5 and .75 to get a range of grams per day. If you are a 120-pound woman, you will need somewhere between 60 and 90 grams of protein per day, and if you are a 180-pound male, you will need between 90 and 135 grams. It may be a good idea to look through these food lists to see how you can meet your protein needs with vegetarian options in the backcountry.

When you are eating servings of meat, poultry, or fish, it is easier to estimate your protein intake, since three ounces provides about 25 grams of protein, compared to plant foods with 3 to 10 grams of protein per average serving. Soy foods are an exception in that a half-cup of soy nuts provides 18.5 grams of protein. If you eat cheese you will get over 10 grams per ounce (plus it will increase the protein profile of any plant foods you eat with it). Remember also, when you are estimating your intake in the backcountry after a long day on the trail, that you will likely want to eat larger servings than the amounts listed in the protein table.

OTHER NUTRIENTS OF CONCERN FOR VEGETARIANS

While people are most concerned about getting enough protein with a vegetarian diet, the nutrients that vegetarians really need to pay attention to include iron, zinc, calcium, vitamin D, and vitamin B_{12}, particularly vegans that eat no animal foods. Iron and zinc are both very important nutrients in the backcountry.

Iron is needed to make new red blood cells to carry oxygen to working muscles, and zinc is important for generating energy and supporting immune function. Both iron and zinc are absorbed better from animal foods than plant sources. We absorb roughly 20 to 30 percent of the heme iron found in meat and other animal foods (except dairy and eggs that are not good sources of iron) and only 2 to 8 percent of the nonheme iron found in plant foods such as beans, lentils, whole or fortified grains, and dark green leafy vegetables. Vitamin C does increase the absorption from plant foods, so making meals that combine vitamin C–rich tomato sauce with pasta and beans is a good choice. This may be a particularly good strategy early on in your backcountry adventure when your body is making new red blood cells to accommodate the increased physical activity or when you are preparing to travel to high altitude.

Zinc is better absorbed from animal foods because the dietary fiber and phytates in whole grains (one of the better plant sources of zinc) interfere with absorption. This may actually be another benefit of using more of the convenient refined grains in the backcountry that contain less fiber and phytates. Dairy foods are well-absorbed sources of zinc, so vegans may need to

Nutritional Yeast

This non-active yeast contains amino acids, some carbohydrate, and very little fat. Nutritional yeast is high in many B vitamins (and often cultivated with the active form of vitamin B_{12}) and has been used by vegans for many years as a nutritional supplement. This special yeast has a cheesy, nutty flavor and is available in either golden colored flakes or a powder. It is commonly used as a substitute for Parmesan cheese on pasta or as a topping for popcorn. Nutritional yeast is a great addition to your backcountry spice kit to flavor foods, plus add some nutrition.

plan more carefully than vegetarians that eat dairy. You should also know that even though warnings for vegetarians regarding iron and zinc appear often, there is no evidence that "well-fed" vegetarians are deficient in iron or zinc more often than meat-eaters.

> ► **Coffee and the tannins in tea can block the absorption of iron and zinc from foods. Drink these beverages between meals to maximize your absorption of these minerals when eating a vegetarian diet.**

The concern with vitamin B_{12} is, once again, more for vegans than other types of vegetarians. This important vitamin, also linked to red blood cell formation as well as nerve tissues, is found naturally only in animal foods unless a product is fortified. While there is some B_{12} in sea plants, sea vegetables, and a few other plant foods, it is not the form of B_{12} that our bodies can use. Nutritional yeast, some cereals, and several other foods geared towards vegetarians are fortified with B_{12}. It also takes a long time to develop a deficiency of B_{12} since we need very small amounts of it and our bodies store it, so if you enter the field with enough B_{12}, it is not likely you will develop a deficiency.

Calcium is also a concern for vegans or other vegetarians who do not eat dairy or calcium-fortified substitutes, since milk and other dairy products are major sources of calcium. Out of the field, this is less of a problem since there are now many juices and different kinds of milk (rice, soy, almond, etc.) with added calcium. Powdered soymilk fortified with calcium is a good backcountry source. Many dark green vegetables such as broccoli, kale, and collard greens are good plant sources, though they contain less calcium per serving than dairy foods. In the field, however, where these foods are not part of your typical backcountry menu, it is more challenging to meet your calcium needs. If you are adventurous and in a place where dandelions grow wild, one cup of raw dandelion greens contains 190 milligrams of calcium (compared to 88 grams for ⅔ cup of broccoli or 300 milligrams for an 8-ounce glass of milk). (See the tables on the following page for nondairy sources of calcium and ideas for adding calcium to your vegetarian meals in the backcountry.)

Vitamin D is another vitamin found only in animal or fortified foods (fatty fish, fortified milk, egg yolk). Vitamin D has long been known for its role in bone health since it is needed to absorb and use calcium. Recently, however, vitamin D has been linked to a variety of important body functions beyond bone health, including muscle growth and strength, chronic inflammation, and immune system function (see the vitamin chapter in section I for more details). The good news is that all of this information is leading to more fortified foods, even some that are not of animal origin like cereals and energy bars.

Ways to Add Calcium Without Dairy

- Add blackstrap molasses to cereals or pancakes (mix with honey, sugar, or pure maple syrup if taste is too bitter).
- Snack on soy nuts, almonds, brazil nuts, sunflower seeds, hazelnuts, raisins, figs, and dates.
- Look for cereals, pancake mixes, and other drink mixes fortified with calcium.
- Make a backcountry salad with dandelion greens—add sesame or sunflower seeds and sliced dried figs for even more calcium.
- Eat quinoa, buckwheat, quick-cooking barley, or brown rice.

Calcium Without Cows

(Nondairy Sources of Calcium)

Food or Beverage*	***Serving Size***	***Milligrams of Calcium***
Milk (for comparison)	1 cup (8 ounces)	300
Soy milk (fortified)	1 cup	200 to 400
Almonds	1/4 cup	80
Blackberries	1/2 cup	23
Blackstrap molasses	1 tablespoon	170
Broccoli, cooked	1 cup	178
Buckwheat pancake mix	1/3 cup	80
Collard greens, cooked	1 cup	148
Corn tortilla (Pepe's)	1 tortilla	100
Dandelion greens	1 cup (raw)	190
Figs	3	81

Food or Beverage*	***Serving Size***	***Milligrams of Calcium***
Flaxseed	3 tablespoons	80
Kale, cooked	1 cup	94
Nutri Grain Waffles, frozen	2	100
Raisins	1/2 cup	40
Refried beans (Rosarita, vegetarian style)	1/2 cup	40
Sardines, canned with bones	3 1/2 ounces	240
Salmon, canned with bones	3 1/2 ounces	237
Seaweed, Arame (many varieties with different amounts of Ca)	1/2 cup	100
Sesame seeds	1 ounce	37
Soy nuts	1/4 cup	60
Tabouli	1/3 cup (dry)	60
Tofu (made with calcium sulfate)	3 ounces	150

*Many other beans, nuts, seeds, and grains contain calcium in varying amounts, as well as fortified juices, cereals, and other products. Look for foods with sesame seeds, almonds, buckwheat, and blue corn (some but not all seem to have more calcium than their white or yellow corn counterparts). Copyright Beyond Broccoli Nutrition Counseling.

FOOD ALLERGY VERSUS INTOLERANCE

There is much confusion about the difference between food allergy and food intolerance. Part of this confusion is a general misunderstanding about the difference between these two conditions.

FOOD INTOLERANCE

There are several reasons food intolerance develops, but the main characteristic that distinguishes intolerance from allergy is that intolerance does not involve an immune response. One example is lactose intolerance that develops when the body does not produce enough of the enzyme lactase needed to properly digest lactose (milk sugar). Sufferers may produce some lactase and may tolerate some amount of dairy without symptoms.

Lactose intolerance is a very common condition worldwide; in the United States, one in nine Americans are estimated to be lactose intolerant, mainly as adults. There is no life-threatening consequence from eating foods with lactose (dairy), but a wide range of unpleasant digestive symptoms are common, such as cramping, bloating, diarrhea, excessive gas, nausea, and stomach pain, as well as occasional headache and fatigue. The symptoms often occur after drinking milk or eating ice cream (or frozen yogurt) and may happen only above a certain amount. There is a lot of individual variability in how people react to dairy foods, even with lactose intolerance. Most cheese is very low in lactose so it may be consumed without ill effects, and the beneficial bacteria in yogurt (regular, not frozen) may predigest some of the lactose, making it tolerable.

There are other foods that may cause digestive or other symptoms in some people. Usually the amount eaten affects the reaction and severity of symptoms. Unfortunately, dehydration, exercise-induced low blood sugar, and other factors in the backcountry can cause similar symptoms, so it is difficult to identify food intolerance based solely on a backcountry experience with food. Another relatively common food intolerance that may be under-diagnosed is fructose, the sugar that occurs naturally in fruit and is processed to make the high fructose corn syrup that is added to many processed foods. Again, because dried fruit is the most common backcountry fruit, and being physically dehydrated can make dried fruit more difficult to digest, experiencing digestive symptoms after eating fruit in the backcountry does not mean you are allergic to or intolerant of fruit. (It probably means you need to drink more water!)

FOOD ALLERGY

According to the American Academy of Allergy, Asthma, and Immunology, a food allergy is the result of an abnormal immune response after eating a food (all other non-immunological responses to foods are intolerance). Basically, with a food allergy your body sees a food as harmful and treats it like a dangerous invader. The allergic response occurs within several minutes to two hours after eating the offending food. These reactions include typical allergy symptoms such as hives, rashes, stuffy or runny nose, itching, swelling, or difficulty breathing. The most severe reaction is anaphylaxis, which is life-threatening and often requires epinephrine or steroids to reverse and treat. The incidence of what some call "true" food allergy is only 1.5 to 2 percent of the general population and slightly higher among children (5 to 7 percent). The most common food allergies include milk, eggs, peanuts, tree nuts, fish, shellfish, soy, and wheat.

Most Common Food Allergens

Milk	Peanuts	Fish	Soy
Eggs	Tree nuts	Shellfish	Wheat

Another reason for the confusion about food allergies is the increase in alternative food allergy tests that are not based on the traditional reactions to IgE antibodies. Alternative tests measure the levels of IgG antibodies (instead of IgE), and the theory is that over time, repeated exposure to foods will increase these antibodies. An abundance of these antibodies may cause digestive system problems such as diarrhea, constipation, bloating, and cramping or nonspecific symptoms (meaning there can be many possible causes) such as headaches, fatigue, and low energy. Unfortunately, these tests are not widely accepted in the medical community due to a lack of adequate scientific evidence that they are accurate. Yet many people that have a history of various digestive or other symptoms and are disillusioned with the current medical system are turning to alternative medicine as a way to address their symptoms. While in many cases this is a positive trend that encourages people to be proactive about their health care, in this instance, it can be a problem.

As other sections of this book have pointed out, backcountry nutrition is challenging enough with so many food factors to consider, such as weight, perishability, ease of preparation, and nutritional value. Dietary restrictions mean food choices are even more limited. The more restrictive a particular diet is, the more difficult it will be to get everything you need nutritionally in the field. Obviously, if you truly have a food allergy, the kind where you swell up and the chance you may not be able to breathe is imminent, you must completely avoid the offending food. If you have been diagnosed by one of the less valid tests that suggest you must eliminate a long list of foods, it may be worth making sure that the food really is a problem before you make your backcountry diet more difficult. You could try an elimination diet where you don't eat the offending food (or foods, if you suspect more than one) for two or three weeks; then slowly reintroduce the food(s) one at a time and record any ill effects.

GLUTEN-FREE DIETS

Gluten is a protein found in wheat (semolina, seitan, spelt, and triticale), rye, barley, and contaminated oats. There is both allergy and intolerance associated with gluten. There are also people who can tolerate spelt, rye, and barley but not other forms of wheat. Wheat-free does not always mean gluten-free, so if it is gluten that is your problem, you must be very careful to read labels.

Celiac disease is a serious intolerance related to an autoimmune response (other autoimmune diseases include type 1 diabetes, multiple sclerosis, and rheumatoid arthritis). With this disease, eating even small amounts of gluten destroys the villi lining the small intestine that aid the absorption of many nutrients. Chronic anemia or early diagnosis of osteopenia may be related to undiagnosed celiac that has caused a chronic malabsorption of nutrients. There is no cure for celiac, and the only treatment is a gluten-free (GF) diet. It is not known if the recent increase of this disease (one in one hundred thirty-three people in the U.S.) is due to better diagnostics or some other factors such as the amount of highly processed wheat consumed.

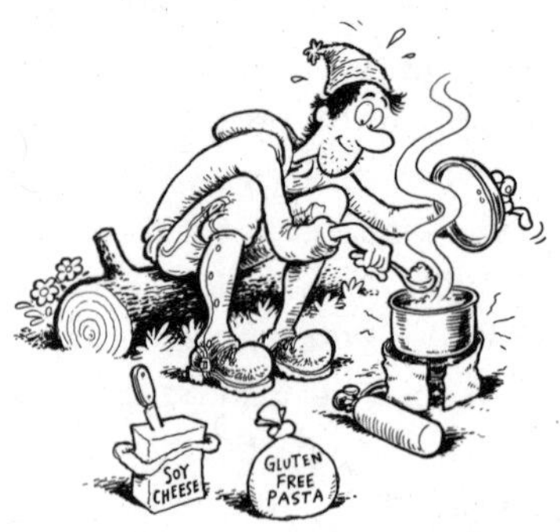

Gluten-free Grains (or Grain Substitutes)

Amaranth
Arrowroot
Beans (there are also many flours made from beans)
Buckwheat (groats, toasted groats or kasha, flour)
Corn (yellow, blue)—whole kernels, popped, corn tortillas, cornmeal
Flaxseed
Garfava
Millet—toast before cooking for added flavor
Nut flours
Oats
Potato
Quinoa ("keen-waah")—cooks in 15 to 20 minutes; eat like rice or breakfast grain
Rice (rice bran)—brown, wild, Red Wehani, Basmati
Sorghum
Soy
Tapioca
Teff

In the backcountry, managing a gluten-free diet is difficult but possible. It requires not mixing foods or utensils (if you use an unwashed knife that someone used to make a PBJ sandwich, you will spread gluten to your food). There are many bread products, such as pita pockets and muffins, made with alternative flours, but most are sold from the freezer case and spoil quickly if not refrigerated. There are pastas, hot cereals, and other mixes made from corn, rice, quinoa, legumes, and buckwheat that are fine for the backcountry. In fact, the rations departments throughout NOLS locations worldwide try to accommodate gluten-free diets in the field. Some of the departments stock GF items. And some of the more remote NOLS locations—where such foods are not readily available—will work with students prior to the trip to adjust individual rations. One positive side to the increase in the number of people diagnosed with celiac is that there are many more GF foods available in regular grocery stores and online (health food stores have always carried a decent selection of GF foods).

The two biggest backcountry nutrition challenges related to a GF diet are getting enough carbohydrates and dietary fiber. It is important to make sure you are keeping up with your glycogen stores with carbohydrate-rich foods. It does take more effort to find GF alternatives, and some of these foods are definitely acquired tastes, so it is a good idea to experiment before you go into the field as much as possible. Many of the alternative grains (though not all) are lower in fiber than wheat, rye, and barley, and many of the products made from these grains are even lower in fiber due to processing. Without fresh fruits and vegetables to add fiber to your meals and snacks, it is important to include beans, legumes, dried fruit, nuts, and seeds to increase the fiber content of your backcountry diet. This will also make sure you are getting some of the vitamins and minerals that are removed during the processing of the alternative grains.

FINAL THOUGHTS FOR THE FIELD

While careful planning and some creativity are needed, it is possible to meet your nutritional needs in the backcountry with a restricted diet. There are more resources than ever before to procure foods without animal products, dairy, wheat, gluten, and any other foods that may cause allergy, intolerance, or psychological aversion. I do think it is important to make sure that you truly have a food allergy before you eliminate a wide range of foods that will make backcountry meal planning more difficult. This holds true for food preferences such as vegetarianism that are pursued for health reasons. You may find that your health is better served in the backcountry with a less restrictive diet.

CHAPTER 12

COMING HOME: NUTRITION AFTER GETTING OUT OF THE FIELD

Take rest; a field that has rested gives a bountiful crop.
—Ovid

Whether you are transitioning out of the backcountry following a big adventure and ready to get back to "real life" or just enjoying a frontcountry fix between trips, there are some nutrition guidelines that can make the adjustment more enjoyable. Throughout this book there has been discussion about the various nutritional tradeoffs that are made in the backcountry due to the many factors that limit food choices. Now it is time to look at the habits you want to take home and those best left in the backcountry.

Nutritional Tradeoffs to Leave in the Backcountry

Packaged and highly processed foods that contain trans fat (partially hydrogenated oils)

Refined grains that make cooking quick, easy, and convenient but lack many important vitamins, minerals, and fiber

Foods high in sodium (salt) that were great to replace the sodium (an important electrolyte) in sweat during long days of backcountry exercise but aren't necessary in everyday life (and may contribute to health risks like high blood pressure)

Less fresh foods—this is realistic in the backcountry but cutting down on fresh foods is not a great nutrition strategy for everyday life

Backcountry Habits to Take Home

Eat more high-fiber foods: legumes, nuts, seeds (adding whole grains as well as fresh fruits and vegetables).

Eat smaller amounts of food throughout the day as needed (rather than three big meals), to keep blood sugar and energy levels steady.

Drink enough fluid to properly hydrate throughout the day.

Eat less saturated fat by enjoying a more plant-based diet (not necessarily a vegetarian diet, just more plant foods than the average frontcountry diet).

Make time to enjoy meals, both the preparation and the eating.

Eat a variety of foods to get the full array of nutrients you need to feel well and stay healthy. (This is easier to do at home, but many people stick to their routines; after a backcountry trip, you may have some new ideas.)

Recognize that small amounts of special treats can be very satisfying (like the chocolate that you parceled out for a week in the backcountry, but would typically last just minutes at your desk!).

In the backcountry, food choices are for immediate performance and survival. There are some very practical reasons for the food choices we make and, though nutrition is important and may be one of the considerations, there are factors that override optimal nutrition with some of the choices. When you come out of the field, your food choices are determined more by personal preference, perhaps convenience, and ideally, nutritional considerations for both immediate and long-term health. Without the limitations of the backcountry and with good health as a goal of eating, there are some adjustments to make when coming out of the field.

BACKCOUNTRY FOOD FANTASIES

I often find myself fantasizing about food. I imagine myself winning the noodle eating contest at the Mongolian restaurant . . . pizza and burgers used to excite me but now it's more to do with things I can't get on or near the Trail.

—Appalachian Trail Through-Hiker

Inevitably, extended trips into the backcountry include some amount of fantasizing about the foods (and beverages) missing

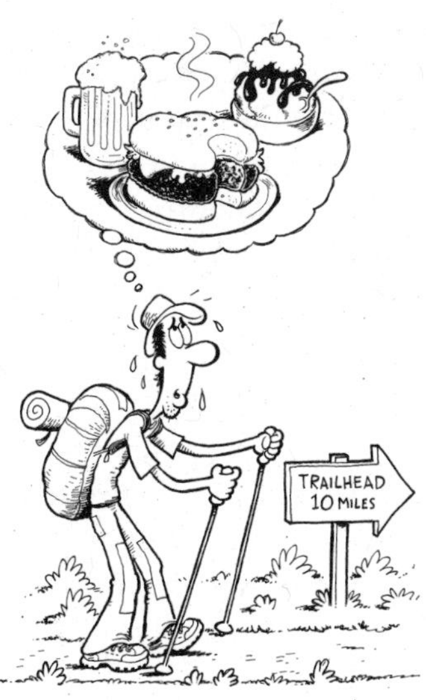

from the menu. Toward the end of the trip it is common to daydream and discuss in which of these foods you will indulge once you get back to civilization. Pizza, ice cream, burgers, fries, and cold beer are common among these wish lists. Of course, healthier fare like fresh salads and fruit are also among the foods most missed during backcountry ventures where these foods are not available.

It is interesting to observe our reaction to food limitations, even when there are enough calories. We are so accustomed to having a wide variety of foods available to us most of the time that, if we don't have access to the types or amounts of food we usually do, it can create psychological stress and affect our moods. Conversely, after a period of relatively limited food supplies, it is typical to have cravings for specific foods. If there is a food shortage during the backcountry adventure, depending upon the degree of the shortage, such as smaller than desired portions or required fasting, you may experience eating binges, preoccupation with food and eating, compulsion to hoard food, or other psychological and emotional responses, following your return. (See chapter 7 for more about food and mood and the psychology of food intake.)

Thankfully, food shortages are not commonplace for most expeditions and readjusting to home life may begin with a longed-for meal but no serious psychological issues. Remember that your body will need time to adapt to changes in the fat and fiber content of your diet. Overdoing high fat, low fiber foods—after an extended period of eating high

► To try to shore up your supply of immune-boosting fruits and vegetables between backcountry trips, think about eating a variety of colors during your front-country reprieve.

fiber, and very likely moderate to low fat backcountry fare—can wreak havoc with your digestive system. Your bowels will also need to readjust to your frontcountry diet, particularly if your everyday food choices are dramatically different than your backcountry menu. In other words, gorging on a huge meal as soon as you get out of the field is not the best idea, even if it seems like the thing to do.

REFUELING BETWEEN TRIPS

Whether you are a backcountry professional, a backcountry student, or a long-distance hiker, these breaks between trips into the field will be an important time to refuel with nutritious fresh foods that are either limited or not available in the backcountry.

AIM TO INCREASE

- Fresh vegetables and fruit to round out the vitamins, minerals, and phytonutrients that are not as abundant in the field
- Fatty fish and ground flaxseed rich in omega-3 fatty acids to boost your immune system (and provide many long-term benefits related to heart and brain health and chronic inflammation)
- Yogurt (or other fermented foods like kefir, miso, and sauerkraut) to add to your colony of beneficial gut bacteria (another way to boost your immune system)
- Whole grains that require more cooking time than you can spare in the backcountry (due to limited fuel, water, or other resources) to keep up your high-fiber intake for digestive health, and to provide a variety of vitamins, minerals, and phytonutrients that boost your immune system (many whole grains provide fuel for the beneficial gut bacteria)
- Animal foods (unless you are a vegetarian) to treat your body to readily available sources of iron, zinc, and vitamin B_{12}

RECALIBRATING YOUR APPETITE

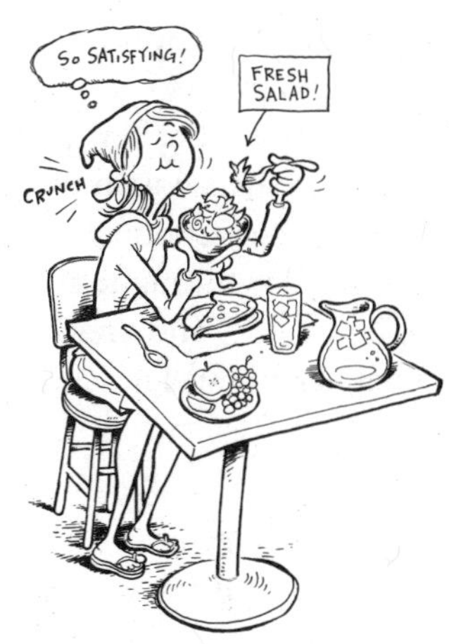

If you venture into the backcountry for extended trips, chances are you also enjoy being physically active when you aren't in the field. Unless you are a professional athlete who gets paid to work out or you don't need to work to support yourself financially, you probably will not be able to maintain the level of physical activity you enjoy in the field, at least not on a daily basis. This means in order to maintain a healthy weight you will have to make some adjustments to the amount of food you eat at home. If you are one of the lucky humans who has maintained the ability to eat only when you are physically hungry and to stop when you have had enough (not full, just sated), the transition from backcountry to home may be naturally smooth.

Many people struggle with this transition, however, because appetite is a complex combination of physiology and psychology. We eat for many reasons, one of which is to fuel ourselves physically, but there are also rituals surrounding meals. There are sensory cues, such as smell, taste, and visual images that entice us to eat with or without physical hunger. As mentioned above, if you felt deprived of certain foods or just craved them while in the backcountry, it is likely you will seek these foods when you get home or between trips. The bottom line is that it may take your body a while to adjust to its need for fewer calories after an extended period of prolonged and often strenuous physical activity.

> ► **Instead of eating large quantities of pizza, washed down with cold beer, and followed by a hot fudge sundae, you could try eating a couple slices of pizza with a big fresh salad, one beer (and lots of water), followed by sharing a dessert. Your digestive system may still struggle but less so.**

It may be helpful to recognize that even if you cannot devote many hours each day to physical activity in your everyday life, focusing on quality versus quantity of exercise can help you balance your calories and maintain more of your lean muscle mass. Continuing to eat smaller (and nutritious) meals and snacks throughout the day can also keep your blood sugar, moods, and energy levels steady, as well as help maintain a healthy weight and lean body mass.

CHAPTER 13 FOR THE BACKCOUNTRY PROFESSIONAL

Expedition planners should not be lulled into a "technology-induced" false sense of security when it comes to planning the nutrition support of an expedition.
—E. Wayne Askew, *Nutrition Support for Expeditions*, 2006

The rise in outdoor-education programs, adventure-travel organizations, and the fact that more adults are choosing to venture into the backcountry means there are a lot of professional educators and guides who spend much of the year in backcountry settings. If you are one of these educators or guides, the information throughout this book should help you to better understand how nutrition can affect, and hopefully enhance, the backcountry experience for you and your clients or students.

The previous chapter includes information about what you can do during the periods of time when you are out of the field. This is your opportunity to eat fresh foods, especially vegetables, fruit, fish, lean meat or poultry, and whole grains, as well as some of the treats you cannot take into the backcountry, like ice cream and pizza. Your personal nutrition out of the field can do a great deal to ensure that you stay healthy in the field.

IN THE FIELD

As with all of the leadership skills you use in the backcountry, applying the principles of good nutrition to yourself is top priority. If you are caring for your own nutritional needs, you are automatically role-modeling good backcountry nutrition for your clients or students. This means getting enough fuel and fluid, spacing your meals and snacks throughout the day to keep your blood sugar and energy levels steady, and eating a variety of foods to make sure you get all of the major nutrients.

If you decide to teach a quick and easy backcountry "Nutrition 101" in the field, here are the top five pearls of nutritional wisdom:

- **Eat and drink often** throughout the day—even if you are working hard or at high altitude and don't feel hungry or thirsty.
- **Never skip** breakfast or dinner.
- **Eat a variety of foods** to make sure you are getting everything you need.
- **Eat and drink more** in the cold, if you are hungry, and after recovery from illness.
- **Eat lots of carbohydrate** foods (and drinks) before, during, and after exercise to fuel brain and muscles.

While these tenets seem pretty basic, it is amazing how many different situations arise that cause backcountry travelers to ignore them. As a backcountry professional, it is likely that your fitness level is significantly higher than the clients and students that you lead into the field. This means that you have more muscle mass than others in your group, and you can store more glycogen (carbohydrate used for quick energy); use fat at a higher intensity level (this allows you to save even more glycogen for your body to use as needed); and potentially have more water storage (glycogen is stored with water).

These physiological adaptations mean you can go longer periods of time without refueling (though you may need more fuel when you do stop) than your less fit students or clients.

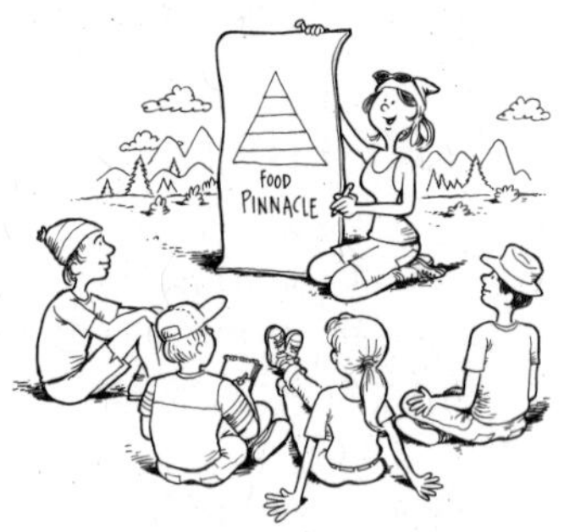

You are also likely to be more acclimated to your environment (hot, cold, or high altitude), or to recognize when you are not and therefore know which steps you need to take while your body adjusts. Your experience enables you to prepare food safely and well (at least to your tastes) and to be aware of your limits with regard to food and water. For example, you may know that even if your blood sugar is dipping a bit, you can nibble on a granola bar and push another hour. What you may not know (at least in the beginning) is the limits of your group.

▸ Remember that female clients and students have less muscle mass than males, even when they are very fit; therefore, they will need to refuel more often. It may improve their self-esteem to learn this is not a sign of weakness but merely reflects a biological gender difference.

Most of the professionals with whom I have had the pleasure of traveling into the backcountry are very attuned to the necessity to make frequent stops for food and water early in the trip while the group is adapting to the environment, building muscle, and learning their needs and limitations. Of course, factors such as impending bad weather or dangerous terrain can override pit stops at times, and the leader must keep group safety first and foremost. It must be emphasized, however, that dehydration and low blood sugar from inadequate fueling can affect one's thinking, strength, coordination, and mood, all of which can endanger that person and possibly the whole group.

One way to plan for situations that don't allow an ideal number of fuel stops is to make sure each group member carries a water bottle with some kind of drink mix that contains carbohydrate calories and, ideally, some electrolytes. The carbohydrates are the most important, though, since this can be enough to keep blood sugar levels steady. Hydration packs are also a good option to allow group members to drink as needed without stopping (though a backup water bottle is recommended in case the hydration pack is punctured, and it is handy for that drink mix, too).

In chapter 10 there are points regarding nutritional concerns with teens going into the backcountry that may also apply to some adult clients or students:

- Unwilling to try new foods—particularly some of the foods needed for key nutrients like protein, iron, and cal-

cium (meal mixes that contain beans and legumes, powdered milk, and alternative nut butters)
- Unaware of symptoms related to dehydration and low blood sugar
- May not eat enough due to body image concerns, not realizing the amount of calories they need to support their backcountry activities (especially women)
- Accustomed to eating only at prescribed times and have trouble with the idea that the backcountry traveler needs to fuel regularly throughout the day
- May not be assertive enough to express needs for food and fluid, perhaps relying on the group leader to initiate such things as rest and fuel stops and eating times
- May not know how to cook, thus cook foods improperly

The difference with adults is that if you can explain the importance of the various nutritional considerations, they are more likely to attempt to make some changes (with teens, who knows, it can have the opposite effect!). The symptoms of dehydration and low blood sugar appear in the next two tables, and more information about these conditions appears in the chapters about water and carbohydrates respectively. In fact, it may help to skim each of the subsequent chapters to find information you may want to share with clients or students in the field.

Symptoms of Hypoglycemia (Low Blood Sugar)		
Dizziness	Fatigue	Fast heartbeat
Confusion	Headaches	Sweating
Disorientation	Extreme hunger	Shaking
Irritability	Anxiety	Impaired vision
Weakness		

Symptoms of Dehydration		
Weakness	Lethargy	Increased heart rate
Headache	Constipation	Decreased urine output
Fatigue	Mental confusion	

NOLS Professionals

During my research for the 2002 *NOLS Nutrition Field Guide*, I discovered that instructors have gone to great lengths to add variety and nutrition (at least in their minds) to the NOLS rations over the past thirty-five years. While fresh fish, energy bars, and hot sauce seem logical, nutritious, and tasty, some of the other trends probably reflect the crazy diet trends of the times in the general population.

The summer 2000 edition of the NOLS alumni newsletter *The Leader* featured an article by Tod Schimelpfenig and his colleagues outlining some of the dietary habits of NOLS instructors from the 1960s through the 1990s. Among the more entertaining gems is the "catfood period" in 1973, featuring dried Little Friskies for an inexpensive source of protein but low in sugar (a twist on the early Atkins diet perhaps?). There were subsequent waves of carnivorous and vegetarian phases, the introduction of energy bars, and experimental periods with cayenne pepper, miso, and Crisco. NOLS Rocky Mountain rations manager and editor of *NOLS Cookery*, Claudia Pearson, mused about "scud missiles," a cheese-filled sausage popular during one of the high fat phases. Given that instructors influence the field diets of at least some students, one can imagine how people out of the field perceived the NOLS rations that were being supplemented with cat food!

Now many NOLS instructors can choose to substitute special items for standard items in order to keep their field menus tailored to their food preferences and, ideally, their nutritional needs. (See appendix C for more information about supplemental foods for NOLS rations.)

SAMPLE BACKCOUNTRY NUTRITION LESSON

If you, as a backcountry professional, understand the importance of nutrition and have some basic nutrition knowledge that applies to the backcountry, you are in a good position to effectively educate your students or clients. One way to engage students or clients about backcountry nutrition is to address some of the nutritional myths and facts that confuse many people, even professionals. Below is a selection of nutrition statements related to backcountry nutrition. Some are myths, some are facts, and some are true in certain situations. The full answers are beneath the list of statements.

Backcountry Nutrition Myths and Facts

Decide if each statement is myth or fact (answers below)

1. You need to rely on protein for energy in the backcountry.
2. Carbohydrates cause you to gain weight and will slow you down in the backcountry.
3. A month in the backcountry is not enough time to develop a vitamin or mineral deficiency.
4. Your body will tell you when it needs food and water.
5. The more protein you eat, the more muscles you build.
6. Antioxidant supplements like vitamins C and E can keep you from getting sick in the backcountry.
7. You need sports drinks to replace electrolytes lost in sweat.
8. The best time to replace your carbohydrate stores is fifteen to thirty minutes after exercise.
9. The more fit you are, the more fat you burn and you don't need as many carbohydrates.
10. It is difficult to get enough protein eating a vegetarian diet.
11. If you are tired in the morning, extra sleep is more important than breakfast.
12. If you are tired when you get to camp and know you are going to bed as soon as possible, it is okay to skip dinner so you don't eat right before bedtime.
13. You can absorb only a certain amount of water at a time so it is best to drink small amounts of fluid throughout the day.
14. Fat is the best source of energy for exercise in the backcountry.

Answers to Backcountry Nutrition Myths and Facts

1. ***You need to rely on protein for energy in the backcountry.***
   Myth. You may need some protein for energy at the end of a long, strenuous day, but protein should not be your primary source of energy in the backcountry. Once your muscle glycogen (stored carbohydrate) is gone, your body may break down muscle to use some of the amino acids from the muscle protein for up to 15 percent of the energy you need, but this process is slow and inefficient. Because protein has many important functions that carbohydrate and fat cannot do, relying on protein for energy is not a good idea.

2. ***Carbohydrates cause you to gain weight and will slow you down in the backcountry.***
   Myth. Carbohydrates are your brain's preferred fuel source and the most efficient, readily available energy when you are working hard or traveling in a hot, cold, or high-altitude environment. Any food you eat in excess of your needs—whether it is high in carbohydrate, protein, or fat—will be stored as fat. Relying on fat and protein to fuel your brain and working muscles in place of carbohydrate will cause you to slow down in the backcountry (or the frontcountry!).

3. ***A month in the backcountry is not enough time to develop a vitamin or mineral deficiency.***
   Fact (if you go into the backcountry well-nourished and take precautions in situations that lead to excessive sweat losses). Some of the water-soluble vitamins that your body doesn't store in large amounts, such as many of the B vitamins and vitamin C, do need to be supplied as you go along. It is possible (at least in theory) to get less than an optimal amount of these vitamins, which could affect your health and performance. However, if you eat a varied diet that includes enough calories, it is unlikely that you will develop a full-blown vitamin or mineral deficiency in a month or even a couple of months. One exception is a deficiency of minerals that act as electrolytes (particularly sodium and potassium) that can be lost in sweat while exercising in the backcountry.

4. ***Your body will tell you when it needs food and water.***
   Myth. It is counterintuitive that there are times when your body does not tell you what it needs, but this is the reality of certain backcountry environments and situations. By the time you are thirsty while exercising, you are already dehydrated. At high altitude, in hot environments, and during strenuous exer-

Backcountry Nutrition Myths and Facts (continued)

cise, your appetite may be suppressed. If you are going into an environment or facing a strenuous day of physical activity, you may need to schedule feedings rather than rely on your body to tell you what it needs. You also need to drink periodically without regard to thirst while you are in the backcountry.

5. ***The more protein you eat, the more muscles you build.***
   Myth. This nutrition myth just won't go away. You do need enough protein to build new muscle, but extra protein does not mean extra muscle. Building muscle requires exercise that stresses the muscle and enough protein to support the process of building muscle. Your body does not store protein per se, and excess protein is stored as fat, just like excess carbohydrate and fat.

6. ***Antioxidant supplements like vitamins C and E can keep you from getting sick in the backcountry.***
   Myth. Antioxidant nutrients like vitamins C and E do play an important role in your immune system function, but there is not compelling evidence that supplements of these vitamins will keep you from getting sick. Vitamin C has been linked to a slightly shorter duration for colds but not to preventing them. Eating a variety of plant foods (dried fruit, vegetables, nuts, seeds, legumes, and grains) that contain these and other antioxidant compounds, along with good backcountry hygiene and safe food handling, are the best strategy for staying well in the backcountry.

7. ***You need sports drinks to replace electrolytes lost in sweat.***
   Myth. If your backcountry adventure involves exercise in extreme climates that generate a lot of sweating, then replacing electrolytes is important. This can be done by consciously including sodium (salt) in your meals and snacks throughout the day and by alternating plain water with some kind of drink mix. If you don't have a sports drink that specifically includes electrolytes, you can add some salt to a regular drink mix that already has some carbohydrate (sugar). You do not need a special sports drink.

8. ***The best time to replace your carbohydrate stores is fifteen to thirty minutes after exercise.***
   Fact. Immediately after a hard workout, your muscles are ready to be replenished, and eating or drinking (or both) a source of carbohydrates with some protein will help this process. If, however, you have severely depleted your glycogen (carbohydrate) stores during a long day of exercise, this

ideal "window" does not replace the need for a carbohydrate-rich dinner, as well as even an additional snack before bedtime or carbohydrates at breakfast prior to exercise.

9. ***The more fit you are, the more fat you burn and you don't need as many carbohydrates.***
   Myth. Increasing fitness does mean you can store more carbohydrate as glycogen (because you have more muscle) and use fat at a higher intensity level. As soon as you begin breathing hard, you are burning more carbohydrate than fat. As you become more fit, you can tolerate more strenuous activity before this happens, meaning you can use fat more than when you were less fit. This does not mean you need fewer carbohydrates, though. In fact, as you build muscle, your metabolism increases and you need more fuel in general. When you are more fit, you may need to eat less often because you will have more glycogen (carbohydrates) stored and can spare these stores by using fat at a higher level of physical activity.

10. ***It is difficult to get enough protein eating a vegetarian diet.***
    Myth. If you eat a variety of plant foods that provide protein throughout the day (legumes, nuts, seeds, and grains) and are meeting your calorie needs, you are probably getting plenty of protein. If you eat some animal foods, such as dairy, eggs, or fish, getting enough protein is even easier. If you are a vegan, you do need to plan a bit more carefully, but it does not have to be difficult to get enough protein. (There are other nutrients more difficult to get from strict vegetarian diets—see chapter 11.)

11. ***If you are tired in the morning, extra sleep is more important than breakfast.***
    Myth. While sleep is important, starting a day in the backcountry without a good breakfast, especially a day that involves a lot of physical activity, is a bad idea. If you begin a day of hiking, climbing, or skiing without eating in the morning, your glycogen stores that fuel your brain already may be half gone just from the fast between dinner and morning. It can take up to twenty-four hours to replenish depleted glycogen stores (in both muscles and liver), so breakfast is an important part of rebuilding your supply from the previous day (or days).

12. ***If you are tired when you get to camp and know you are going to bed as soon as possible, it is okay to skip dinner so you don't eat right before bedtime.***

Backcountry Nutrition Myths and Facts (continued)

Myth. At the end of a strenuous day when you get to camp and want to climb into your sleeping bag more than anything else, you need to realize that skipping dinner will affect how you feel and perform the next day. Eating a meal close to bedtime can affect the quality of your sleep and how well you digest your meal, so keeping it light in protein, fat and fiber, but rich in carbohydrates, is a good strategy. Even if you have something as light as a package of ramen noodles with some kind of bread or crackers on the side and some drink mix, you will perform better the next day than if you skip dinner altogether.

13. ***You can only absorb a certain amount of water at a time, so it is best to drink small amounts of fluid throughout the day.***
Fact. Your body can absorb 20 to 30 milliliters of fluid per minute, but it can lose up to 50 milliliters per minute when exercising in the heat (or other situations that cause major water losses through sweat). Sipping water (and other fluids) throughout the day will maximize how much your body absorbs.

14. ***Fat is the best source of energy for exercise in the backcountry.***
Myth. Fat is the most concentrated source of energy, providing nine calories per gram compared to just four calories per gram for carbohydrates and protein. You can also store enough fat to fuel several weeks of energy needs, compared to stored carbohydrates that will last a few hours (or less) and no stored protein (except as precious muscle that you don't want to break down for energy unless you have no choice). The caveats here are that you need some carbohydrate to effectively burn fat for fuel, and you need enough oxygen to burn fat. So, when you are huffing and puffing up a huge hill or just trying to set up your tent at high altitude, you are relying more on your stored carbohydrate than fat. Ultimately, fat is an important fuel source in the backcountry. However, your ability to store large amounts of fat compared to carbohydrate, and the need for more oxygen (and some carbohydrate) to burn fat efficiently, shifts the focus to carbohydrates as the most important fuel source in the backcountry.

APPENDIX

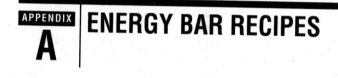

A ENERGY BAR RECIPES

There is no nutritional magic in so-called "energy" bars. Compared to what you can make in your own kitchen, they are simply conveniently packaged with a longer shelf life and often have a more durable texture—and for this you pay more money. Some of these bars tout vitamins, minerals, phytonutrients, and herbs purported to enhance your sports performance or give you more energy. The fact that there is no scientific evidence to back these claims goes largely unnoticed, and eager adventurers fork over a couple of bucks for each bar and hope for the best.

There are lots of ways to make less expensive and more nutritious energy bars at home or in the field. In the following pages you will find two such recipes: the first is a basic recipe that can be made at home before you leave for the field, and the second is a backcountry recipe, Katie's No-Bake Energy Nuggets, from *NOLS Cookery*.

Homemade Energy Bars

This recipe began as an oatmeal cookie recipe and evolved with less sugar (replaced with more nutritious dried fruit) and a better fat profile (nuts and peanut butter) to add protein and nutrients. This makes a delicious treat for sustained energy. Be creative with this recipe by using a variety of fruit, nuts, and grains (millet, quinoa, or amaranth can be used in place of some of the oats) in order to suit your taste and texture preferences.

INGREDIENTS

$^1/_2$ cup brown sugar
1 egg
$^1/_4$ cup peanut butter
2 tsp. vanilla extract
$^1/_2$ cup apple juice (unsweetened)
1 cup whole wheat flour
$^1/_2$ cup dried fruit (raisins, apricots, or dried cranberries)
$^1/_2$ cup chopped nuts (walnuts, almonds, or peanuts)
$^1/_2$ cup semisweet or dark chocolate chips
1 cup quick cooking oats
$^1/_2$ cup wheat germ
$^1/_2$ tsp. baking powder
$^1/_2$ tsp. baking soda
$^1/_4$ tsp. salt
$^1/_2$ tsp. ground cinnamon

Preheat oven to 350°. First mix dry ingredients in one bowl; next mix wet ingredients with "goodies" (chocolate chips, raisins, nuts, etc.) in another bowl; then combine. Spread batter over a lightly greased cookie sheet about $^1/_2$ to $^3/_4$ inch thick. Use a spoon dipped in hot water to press the batter into the sheet to make firm bars. Bake for 10 to15 minutes. Allow pan to cool completely before cutting into bars. (Bars can be refrigerated or frozen prior to your backcountry journey for a longer shelf life.) ***Makes about 20 small bars.***

Nutrition Information (based on raisins and walnuts for fruit and nuts): 1 bar = 140 calories, 20g carbohydrate, 5g protein, 6g fat, 2g fiber

Katie's No-Bake Energy Nuggets

This is an awesome field recipe contribution from my dietitian colleague and friend Katie Wewer, a fellow graduate from the University of Utah's Division of Nutrition. Katie collaborated on the fifth edition of *NOLS Cookery,* teaches wilderness nutrition at the University of Utah, and is an avid backcountry traveler.

INGREDIENTS

1/2 cup sunflower seeds and/or chopped nuts
1 cup raisins, craisins, or small dried fruit pieces
1/2 cup hydrated granola (combined with 2 cups warm water to hydrate granola) or 1/2 cup cooked brown/white rice
1/2 cup nut butter (peanut, almond, or cashew)
1/2 cup powdered milk
1/2 cup honey
1 cup dried regular or instant oatmeal
1 tsp. cinnamon
few drops of vanilla
1/4 to 1/2 cup whole wheat flour

Mix all ingredients except flour together and stir. The mixture will be sticky. Gradually add flour until the mixture becomes less sticky. Let mixture set in a cool place (in the snow, under a shaded tree or rock, or in a stream) for 15 to 20 minutes or until the ingredients bind together. Pinch off small amounts and roll into 2-inch nuggets. Store in a sealed container or plastic bag. These energy nuggets are very dense, so you probably need to eat only one at a time. Keep these divine little edibles as cool as possible. Eat within one to two days. ***Makes 30 bite-size nuggets.***

Nutrition information: 4 nuggets = 749 calories, 111g carbohydrate, 23g protein, 29g fat, 11g fiber.

APPENDIX B

BACKCOUNTRY NUTRITION PINNACLE

The Backcountry Nutrition Pinnacle is an adaptation of the USDA Food Pyramid designed to consider the nutritional realities of backcountry travel and living. The categories are similar, but the pinnacle places a particular emphasis on water and carbohydrates to fuel backcountry exercise and other activities. The fruit and vegetable groups are expanded to include the many plant foods that fit into a backcountry pantry and offer similar nutrients, phytonutrients, and dietary fiber that are available from the USDA fruit and vegetable group. The protein group includes dairy.

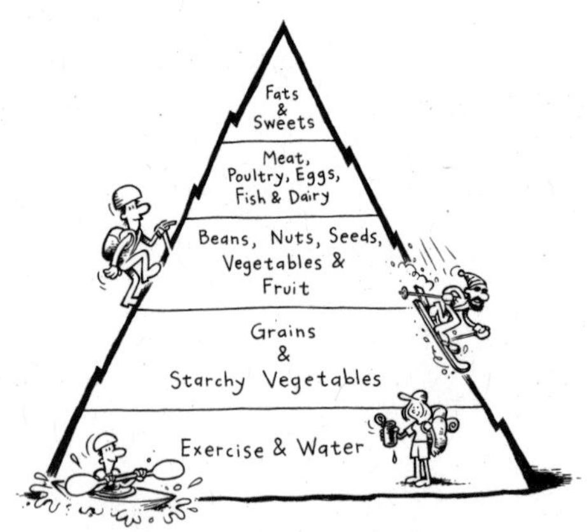

1. WATER AND EXERCISE

At the base of the backcountry pinnacle are exercise and water. Water is the most important nutrient for both survival and optimal nutrition in the backcountry. Most days in the field a person will require a minimum of two to three quarts of water and a variety of other fluids. Water can be supplemented with tea, drink mixes, hot cocoa, and soups to meet the higher fluid needs for exercise in the backcountry.

Many nutritionists recommend limiting beverages that contain caffeine, alcohol, excessive sugar, or carbonation surrounding exercise. However, current research on the effects of these beverages on hydration status is not clear. Moderation is probably the best rule of thumb, given that excessive amounts of caffeine can cause the jitters and stomach upset, alcohol can impair judgment and motor skills, and excessive sugar is a poor nutritional choice. Adding some sugar (or other sweetener, such as honey or maple syrup) can help you get enough carbohydrates during long days of exercise, and salty beverages may be helpful when exercising in the heat.

2. GRAINS AND STARCHY VEGETABLES

A combination of whole and processed grains and starchy vegetables is an appropriate base of nutrition for high levels of physical activity. These foods also tend to be quick and easy to prepare in the backcountry. This group is high in carbohydrate, the nutrient most easily converted to energy and your brain's preferred fuel source. While whole grains contain more vitamins, minerals, and dietary fiber than refined grains, compromises must be made in the backcountry due to available fuel, water, and preparation time.

In addition to carbohydrates, this group contains B vitamins and iron, which are essential for energy production, immunity, and a healthy nervous system. The grains are also a source of vegetable proteins that combine with beans, nuts, and seeds to make complete proteins necessary for building and repairing body cells.

Number of servings: Include grains or starchy vegetables at most meals and snacks. Serving sizes vary and are outlined below.

Serving sizes: $\frac{1}{2}$ cup cooked grains/starchy vegetable (rice, pasta, potatoes, etc.), 1 slice bread, $\frac{1}{2}$ bagel, 2 cups cooked popcorn, and $\frac{1}{4}$ to $\frac{1}{2}$ cup of snack mixes.

Sources: pasta, bread, cereal, rice, couscous, flour, cornmeal, pancake mix, bulgur, popcorn, potatoes, crackers, and many of the snack mixes.

3. VEGETABLES, FRUIT, BEANS (LEGUMES), NUTS, AND SEEDS

Out of the field, fruits and vegetables form a separate group, and five to nine servings a day from this group is recommended. In the backcountry, we often rely heavily on smaller amounts of dried fruits and vegetables, and five servings each day is not always possible. So, the pinnacle includes vegetables, fruits, beans, nuts, and seeds in one large group. These plant foods are all sources of carbohydrates, dietary fiber, and many of the same vitamins, minerals, and phytonutrients (beneficial plant compounds) found in the USDA pyramid groups that contain these foods.

In addition to contributing carbohydrates, the expanded vegetable group provides protein and healthy fats (beans, nuts, and seeds). This group also supplies the antioxidant vitamins A, C, and E, as well as many of the B vitamins and other minerals that are important for resistance to infections, wound healing, muscle tissue growth and repair, and overall healthy cells.

Number of servings: five to eight per day

Serving sizes: 1 cup fresh fruit or vegetables (1 to 2 tablespoons

dried), 1 ounce nuts or seeds, 2 tablespoons nut butter, $\frac{1}{4}$ to $\frac{1}{2}$ cup rehydrated hummus, soup, chili mixes, etc.
Sources: dried or fresh vegetables, wild greens, garlic, tomato powder, vegetable soups, peas in oriental mix, fresh or dried fruit, wild berries, nuts, peanut butter, seeds, bean flakes, dehydrated beans, hummus, veggie burger mix, chili mix, and lentil soup.

4. FISH (WHEN AVAILABLE), DAIRY, POULTRY, MEAT, AND EGGS

This group is a combination of the groups in the USDA pyramid that feature calcium and protein. Milk powder (cow or soy), cheese, and powdered egg are common backcountry foods also high in animal protein. Calcium found in milk and cheese is important for the structure of bones and teeth as well as muscle contraction, blood clotting, and enzyme activation. In addition to calcium, milk and cheese provide the B vitamin riboflavin, an important nutrient for carbohydrate metabolism and skin health.

Other animal proteins such as jerky, summer sausage, canned chicken or tuna, and fresh fish caught from lakes and streams may supplement backcountry rations in this group. These foods are not necessary in large amounts or required daily to meet nutritional needs. Beans, legumes, nuts, and seeds also contribute to protein needs and may replace the options in this group. Calcium, iron, and zinc are not easily replaced with other vegetable sources, so careful planning is required for strict vegetarian diets that omit this food group entirely.
Number of servings: one to two servings per day (or less)
Serving size: 1 ounce cheese; 8 ounces milk; 3 ounces fish, poultry, or meat; 1 egg (or powdered equivalent).
Sources: powdered milk (cow or soy), cocoa, all cheeses, cheesecake and pudding mixes, summer sausage, jerky; fresh, canned, or dried fish; canned chicken; or powdered eggs.

5. FATS AND SWEETS

Fats and sweets appear at the top of both the Food Guide Pyramid and the Backcountry Nutrition Pinnacle because our bodies need these in the smallest amounts from a nutritional standpoint. In the Pinnacle, this group includes added vegetable oil or margarine used sparingly for cooking or as a condiment.

Other types of fat appear in both the protein and vegetable groups. These fats are not part of the use-sparingly group because they are more beneficial for health; they include the essential fats in fish and nuts, or they are accompanied by important nutrients such as the calcium and B vitamins in dairy foods.

There are certain foods, such as trail snacks or chocolate and desserts that are "sweets" but appear in other categories of the pinnacle as well because they provide some protein, carbohydrate, and other nutrients. While it is still recommended to use these foods sparingly for optimal nutrition, in the backcountry we use the carbohydrates and added calories from fat in sweet foods to support our high activity level.

In addition to making foods more palatable in the backcountry, the fats and sweets at the top of the pinnacle also can provide a psychological boost on the trail or at the end of a rigorous day of physical activity. Again, nutrition recommendations out of the field generally do not include using food as a reward, but in the field this can be appropriate.

Number of servings: use sparingly and strategically

Serving size: varies with each product, but typically 1 teaspoon is a serving for added fats (oil or butter).

Sources: vegetable oil or margarine, candy, chocolate, snack mixes, sauce mixes, drink mixes, cocoa, summer sausage, pudding, and cheesecake.

APPENDIX C

NOLS STANDARD RATIONS ITEMS AND BULK RATIONING SYSTEM

This is a list of standard ration items at NOLS. Some items vary among NOLS locations due to availability of foods and the types of courses issued from the branch. Throughout NOLS, rations departments are working to source foods locally and organically when possible and to provide foods for special dietary needs. While all NOLS branches do their best to accommodate special dietary needs, remote locations may not have access to special foods such as gluten-free grains or dairy substitutes.

Below are the basic rations found throughout the school, with exceptions that are not widely available preceded by an asterisk (*). Following the table is some information about additional foods provided by specific NOLS branches, as well as a brief overview of the bulk rationing system used by NOLS as they issue food to courses.

Standard Ration Items at NOLS

Item	*Serving size*	*Calories*	*Fat (g)*	*Protein (g)*	*Carb (g)*	*Fiber (g)*	*Sodium (mg)*	*Vit A (RE)*	*Calcium (mg)*	*Iron (mg)*	*Vit C (mg)*
Almonds, unblanched	12–15	93	8.5	2.8	2.9	<1	24	—	38	0.7	tr
Bagel (plain)	1	187	1	7	36	2	363	—	50	2.43	—
Black beans, instant	1/3 cup	160	1.5	7	29	10	310	40	60	2.7	—
Brownie mix	1/4 cup	160	7	2	22	<1	140	—	—	0.72	—
Brown sugar	1 Tbs.	52	—	—	13.4	—	3.4	—	11	0.4	—
Bulgur	100 grams	354	1.5	8	76	11	—	—	23	7.8	—
*Candy, hard	2 pcs	60	—	—	16	—	10	—	—	—	—
Cashews, roasted and salted	6-8 nuts	84	7	2.6	4.4	0.2	2	15	6	0.6	—
Cereal, Nutty Nuggets	1/2 cup	170	1	6	38	5	210	250	—	14.4	—

Cereal, *Perky's Nutty Rice	$^{3}/_{4}$ cup	210	1.5	4	46	2	110	—	—	—	—
Cheese, Jack	1 oz. (1-inch cube)	110	9	7	—	—	180	60	200	—	—
Cheese, cheddar	1 oz.	120	10	7	—	—	180	80	200	—	—
Cheese cake	38 grams	160	4	3	28	—	300	—	150	—	—
Cheese sauce, alfredo and cheese	$^{1}/_{4}$ cup (12 g mix + water)	60	3	1	5	—	290	—	20	—	—
*Chili mix	$^{1}/_{4}$ cup	100	1	5	10	3	560	200	60	1.8	4.8
Chocolate chips	33 pieces	70	4	<1	10	<1	—	—	—	0.36	—
Cider mix, Alpine Cider by Krusteaz	8 oz. (fluid)	80	—	—	19	—	20	—	66.4	0.14	88
Cocoa	2 Tbs.	110	1.5	2	23	1	150	—	100	0.72	1.2
Cornmeal	$^{1}/_{4}$ cup	110	1	2	23	5	11	10	—	0.9	—

Standard Ration Items at NOLS (continued)

Item	*Serving size*	*Calories*	*Fat (g)*	*Protein (g)*	*Carb (g)*	*Fiber (g)*	*Sodium (mg)*	*Vit A (RE)*	*Calcium (mg)*	*Iron (mg)*	*Vit C (mg)*
Couscous	$^1/_4$ cup	200	—	7	40	3	5	—	20	0.72	—
Cracker mix, Fiesta	1 oz. (28 g)	120	6	—	10	1	200	—	—	—	—
Crackers, animal	5 pieces	43	0.9	0.7	8.0	Tr	30	13	5.0	tr	—
Crackers, Wheat Thins	16 pieces	130	4	3	21	1	240	—	—	1.1	—
Crackers, whole grain *Dr. Kracker	25 grams (1 flat-bread)	100	4	5	11	3	190	—	30	1	—
Cream of wheat	3 Tbs. (dry)	120	—	3	25	1	90	—	100	9	—
Cup of soup, chicken	packet	60	1	3	10	—	590	—	—	0.36	—
Cup of soup, tomato or veggie	packet	90	1	20	<1	<1	510	40	100	—	3.6

Dried fruit, mixed	1/4 cup (40 g)	100	—	2	24	3	25	135	—	7.2	1.8
*Drink mix†	5 tsp.	80	—	—	20	—	20	—	—	—	60
Egg, powdered	18.9 g (1 egg)	96.5	5	6	7	—	101	—	23	—	—
*Falafel	1/4 cup	120	2	7	21	6	370	—	40	2.7	1.2
Fig bar	1 cookie	160	3	1	31	1	110	—	20	0.7	—
Flour, white	1 cup	419	1	12	88	3	2	—	17	5.3	—
Flour, whole wheat	1 cup	406	2	15	87	15	6	—	41	4.6	—
*Fruit bars	1	130	2.5	1	28	<1	75	—	—	0.72	—
Garlic, fresh clove	1 (3 g)	4	<1	<1	1	<1	0.05	—	—	0.05	—
*Granola bars	1	190	10	2	24	1	65	—	20	0.36	—
Grits	3 Tbs.	100	—	—	22	2	—	—	1	0.81	—
Hash browns	2/3 cup	100	—	2	22	2	25	—	—	0.36	4.8
*Lentil soup mix	2/3 cup (dry)	210	1	17	36	19	620	200	80	3.6	—

Standard Ration Items at NOLS (continued)

Item	Serving size	Calories	Fat (g)	Protein (g)	Carb (g)	Fiber (g)	Sodium (mg)	Vit A (RE)	Calcium (mg)	Iron (mg)	Vit C (mg)
Malt balls	5 pieces	210	12	2	25	<1	35	20	80	0.36	—
Margarine	1 Tbs.	100	11	—	—	—	99	471	2.8	—	—
Milk, powdered	1 oz. (dry)/ 1 cup	100	—	10	15	—	150	—	350	—	1.2
Nutritional yeast	1 Tbs.	48	0.8	5	—	8	—	—	—	—	—
Oats, rolled	1 cup	145	2	6	25	4	25	4	19	1.59	—
Oats, instant	1 pkt.	103	1.7	4	18	3	283	449	161	6	—
Orange drink mix†	5 tsp.	80	—	—	20	—	20	—	—	—	60
Pancake mix	100 grams (~3/4 cup dry mix)	346	2.7	11	68.7	2	1384	—	460	5.4	—
Pasta, bowtie	3/4 cup (dry)	203	1	8	41	1	26	—	20	2.7	2.4
Pasta, macaroni	3/4 cup (dry)	210	1	7	41	2	—	—	—	1.8	—
Peanuts, honey roasted	1/4 cup	220	18	8	9	3	140	—	40	1.4	—

Peanuts, salted and roasted	1.5 oz. (~1/4 cup)	266	21	10	9	3.4	342	—	23	0.95	—
Peanuts, *yogurt	15 pieces	160	9	3	14	1	11	—	—	—	—
Peanut butter	2 Tbs.	200	16	7	6	2	140	—	—	0.72	—
Peas, dried	9 g	30	—	2	6	1	—	520	45	0.4	12
Peppers, dried mix	9 g	30	—	1	6	1	10	2,100	10	0.6	200
Potato pearls	1/2 cup (120 g)	73	4	2	15	1.4	248	—	22	0.3	3.1
Pretzels	20 pieces	110	1	2	23	2	590	—	—	1.08	—
Pretzels, peanut butter filled	11 pieces	160	7	4	18	1	160	—	—	1.4	—
Pretzels, *yogurt	7 pieces	190	8	2	30	—	140	—	20	0.36	—
Raisin bran	1 cup	170	1	4	42	7	280	150	20	4.5	—
Raisins	1 cup	435	1	5	115	5	17	1	71	3.02	5
*Raisins, choc. covered	1/4 cup	220	9	3	33	2	25	100	60	0.72	—

Standard Ration Items at NOLS (continued)

Item	Serving size	Calories	Fat (g)	Protein (g)	Carb (g)	Fiber (g)	Sodium (mg)	Vit A (RE)	Calcium (mg)	Iron (mg)	Vit C (mg)
Raisins, yogurt	16 pieces	135	6	1	22	<1	10	—	—	—	—
Ramen noodles	1/2 pkg.	180	7.0	4	26	<1	800	—	—	1.4	—
Refried beans	3 oz.	117	3.9	5	16	6.5	315	—	25	1.6	—
Rice, white	1 cup	161	<1	3	35	1	500	—	13	1	—
*Salmon, wild	2 oz.	60	2	10	—	—	280	—	—	0.36	—
*Sesame sticks	1 oz. (28 g)	160	11	3	13	<1	48	—	40	0.36	—
Snack mix, Gardetto's	1/2 cup	150	6	3	20	1	310	—	—	0.72	—
*Soup base, chicken, beef, or veggie	1 Tbs.	31	1.4	1.7	3	Tr	3591	2	26	0.1	—

Soy nuts, roasted	1 cup	453	24	37	30	3.6	4	220	138	4.5	2.2
Summer sausage***	3 oz.	240	19.5	13.5	1.5	—	1035	—	30	—	—
Sunflower seed kernels	1/4 cup	205	18	8	7	2	10	2	42	2.4	1.0
Tomato powder	100 grams	303	2.2	11.5	68	3	30	13100	85	7.8	239
Tortilla, flour	1 (8 inch)	115	2	3	20	1	169	—	44	1.2	—
*Trail mix, Gulch Mix**	1/2 cup	410	27	12	33	5	140	—	80	1.4	—
Tuna***	3 oz.	100	1.5	20	—	1	360	0.36	—	—	—
Vegetables, dried mix	9 g	30	—	1	7	0.5	10	800	15	0.4	3
Vegetable oil, canola	1 Tbs.	120	14	—	—	—	—	—	—	—	—

† The NOLS drink mixes that are referred to throughout the book are called Sahara Burst, and the flavors issued include orange, lemonade, and fruit punch.

**This is an estimated analysis of the Gulch Mix trail mix issued by NOLS Rocky Mountain. (This estimate assumes equal parts of each ingredient and uses items available in the nutritional database—the actual nutritional breakdown may vary considerably depending on who mixes it!) Gulch Mix contains the following: soy nuts, peanuts, honey-roasted peanuts, butterscotch chips, roasted/salted almonds, cashew pieces, and plain and peanut M&Ms.

***Tuna and summer sausage are standard issue for NOLS Alaska and special ration items used for some winter courses from NOLS Rocky Mountain.

SPICE KITS

Small: Salt, pepper, baking yeast, garlic granules, Spike, cinnamon, Italian seasoning (oregano and basil mix), baking powder, soy sauce, hot sauce, and oil
Large: Small kit, plus chili powder, cumin, cayenne, curry powder, vanilla, and vinegar

TRANS FAT

When reviewed for trans fat content (as partially hydrogenated oils), nearly all of the NOLS standard ration items were below the .5 grams per serving that allows manufacturers to declare zero grams trans fat. Rather than add another column, here are the items that still contain more than .5 grams per serving: margarine, Gardetto's snack mix, and cheese sauce.

NOLS rations departments are currently in search of a suitable substitute for margarine that fits the needs for weight, perishability, and cost. Many instructors opt to take butter and/or olive oil into the field, a good choice given the fact that they are relying on these foods for several months of the year. This is not a perfect solution for the general field rations, though, since both of these items spoil faster than margarine, require different packaging (plastic containers for the oil), and are considerably more expensive. NOLS Rocky Mountain is currently testing a European blend of butter and palm oil.

NOLS ROCKY MOUNTAIN

NOLS Rocky Mountain is located in Lander, Wyoming—also home of NOLS International Headquarters—and issues courses year-round. The rations department (affectionately known locally as the Gulch) also sells bulk foods to the local community, so there is a wide selection of additional foods available to accommodate both special dietary needs and personal preferences.

Below is a list of additional bulk foods that are available for instructors to use as substitutions to their rations or to accommodate special dietary needs on courses, as well as for anyone else who would like to purchase them as supplemental foods.

GENERAL

Dried fruit (blueberries, cranberries, mangoes, cherries, apples, figs, dates, and apricots, purchased in organic form when possible)
Instant soups: corn chowder and split pea
Miso

GRAINS AND LEGUMES

Amaranth
Basmati rice, white or brown
Brown rice, short- or long-grain
Lentils, red
Millet
Organic oatmeal
Quinoa
Spelt flour
Steel cut oats, organic
Tabouli
Tempeh
Whole rye flour, organic
Wild rice

NUTS AND SEEDS

Almonds, raw
Cashew pieces, raw
Flaxseeds, blonde and whole
Hazelnuts
Mixed nuts
Nut butters, almond and organic peanut
Pecans
Soy nuts

Tahini, sesame seed butter
Tamari pumpkin seeds
Walnuts

DAIRY-FREE
Lisanatti brand almond cheese (herb, mozzarella, pepper jack, and cheddar)
Soy milk (powdered chocolate, vanilla, and plain)

GLUTEN-FREE (GF)
Almond cheese
Almond Nut-thins crackers
Annie Chinns rice noodles
Baking flour
Bread sticks, sesame and Glutino
Breakfast bars, Glutino
Breakfast cereals, Glutino
Brownie mix
Corn bread mix
Glad corn
Muffin and scone mix
Polenta mix
Pretzels, Glutino
Quick mix, Gluten Free Pantry
Quinoa
Rice pasta, several types
Sea vegetable salad
Thai Kitchen soups and rice noodles

NOLS ALASKA

NOLS Alaska is a remote and seasonal base that is not able to source some of the foods available in the Lower 48. They must order only what they need since they cannot store excess food during the off-season months. NOLS Alaska does accommodate special diets with enough advanced notice for special-order foods. The kayaking courses take more fresh foods (and some canned fruit) than backpacking and mountaineering courses. They do supply most of the NOLS standard rations, plus the following foods:

Apricots, dried
Banana chips
Basil
Broccoli 3-cheese soup
Candy bars
Carrot cake mix
Carrots, fresh
Cashews
Cheerios
Chicken noodle soup
Cream cheese
Gingerbread mix
Grapenuts
Grits
Jelly beans
Jerky
Minestrone
Muffin mix
Mushrooms, dried shiitake
Oil, olive-canola blend
Onions, fresh
Oranges, fresh
Parmesan cheese
Peaches, canned
Pears, canned
Pilot bread, hard tack (unsalted cracker)
Potatoes, fresh
Raisin Bran
Snack mix, Alaskan (peanuts, raisins, M&Ms, almonds, cashews, and salt)
Snack mix, Barcelona (mostly dried fruit)
Snack mix, Celebration (rice crackers, peanuts, sesame sticks, almonds, cashews, and salt)
Summer sausage

Sunflower seeds
Tortillas, corn and flour
Tuna, cans and pouches

NOLS PATAGONIA

NOLS Patagonia is one of the school's international bases, located in Coyhaique, Chile. There are many rations items that reflect the Chilean culture. NOLS Patagonia does accommodate allergies and vegetarian diets, but is not able to source gluten-free foods. Below are some standard items unique to this branch:

Cornflower (Chuchoca)
Cream Cheese
Dried fruit (papaya, dates, apricots, apples, bananas, prunes, tropical mix, and figs)
Dried onions
Dried tomatoes
Granola
Green tea
Hobby and Prestigio (chocolate candy bars)
Honey
Manjar (a sweetened milk type of jam)
Mantecol (peanut type nougat)
Maté
Miso
Oil
Popcorn
Quinoa
Lentils, red and brown
Rice noodles
Salami
Smoked turkey
Soy meat (textured vegetable protein, or TVP)
Soy milk

Tofu
Tortellini
Tuna
Vanilla
Walnuts
Wheat berries

NOLS SOUTHWEST

NOLS Southwest is headquartered in Tucson, Arizona, and is able to provide many of the same standard items as NOLS Rocky Mountain due to the location. They, too, are able to accommodate special dietary needs. Below are some additional foods included in the standard rations:

Banana nut muffin mix
Blueberry muffin mix
Dried pineapple
Goldfish crackers
Granola
Grits
Hummus
Quinoa
Summer sausage
Veggie pasta

NOLS YUKON

NOLS Yukon, based in Whitehorse, Yukon Territory, Canada, generally issues the majority of foods found on the standard rations list. They accommodate special diets as much as they are able; being so remote, this usually requires that students or staff contact them ahead of time to give them a stipend for foods necessary for their particular diet. Recently, NOLS Yukon has ordered a small to moderate supply of nut-allergy and lactose-issue food items. Before this addition, the branch had been primarily a canoe-based program where weight is not an issue or concern. As their course mix changes, however, they plan to acquire more hiking-friendly food items.

NOLS TETON VALLEY

Located in Driggs, Idaho, NOLS Teton Valley is the base for most of NOLS's winter courses and 14- and 15-year-old Adventure Courses. They are able to accommodate students and instructors with allergies and dietary restrictions and have been able to work with dairy, gluten, tree nut, and peanut allergies in the past. In some cases, they'll ask the student to bring supplements to assist in making sure they are maintaining sufficient nutrition in the field. With an eye to lightweight options, they do plan to revamp their spice kits in the future to reduce weight and cater to specific course and age group preferences. In addition to most of the standard NOLS rations items, NOLS Teton Valley also issues the following items:

Granola
Breakfast cereals (Grapenuts, Raisin Bran, Frosted Mini Wheats, and Muesli)
Crystalized ginger
Fantastic World Foods' Nature's Burger veggie and whole grain burger mix
Ginger snaps
Gingerbread mix
Hummus mix
Snickers
Soy milk powder

Winter specific
Bacon
Tater tots
Tempeh

Summer specific
Fresh fruit
Fresh vegetables (carrots, potatoes, onions, and garlic)

NOLS PACIFIC NORTHWEST

NOLS Pacific Northwest (PNW) is based in Conway, in the heart of Washington State's agriculturally-rich Skagit Valley. NOLS PNW's primarily vegetarian rations include a wide variety of foods, similar to those at other branches. They work on a case-by-case basis with students to accommodate special dietary needs and have successfully created rations to accommodate lactose intolerant, wheat and gluten intolerant, tree nut allergic, celiac, and vegan students. Additional foods in the PNW rations include:

Almond cheeses
Bagels, cinnamon raisin
Butter
Cheese (Parmesan, pepper jack, and mozzarella)
Dried mixed veggies
Dried peas and carrots
Flours, organic whole wheat and white
Gingerbread mix
Granolas (Rainforest Crunch, Pumpkin Flax Plus, Cranberry/Orange, Apple/Cinnamon)
Hummus base
Lentils
Muesli
Olive oil
Orzo
Pancake mix, multigrain
Pasta, veggie spiral and spinach twisty
Popcorn
Quinoa
Rice, brown and Jasmine

Soy milk powder
Spice cake mix
Teas
Thai Kitchen instant rice noodle soups (gluten free)
Tortillas, mixed corn and flour
Tuna and salmon packets
Vegetable bouillon

NOLS PNW also supplies all NOLS India courses, including both fall and spring semesters. Approximately 40 percent, by weight, of India course rations are purchased in India. Ration items bought in India include Muesli; white and whole wheat flours; sugar; powdered milk; cocoa; peanut butter; lentils; white and brown rice; spiral, macaroni, and penne pastas; all cheeses; oil; and several Indian spices to supplement the NOLS spice kit. India's Garwhal Mountaineering course requires a special high altitude ration that includes items not typically found in other PNW rations. These items are purchased in the States and include such foods as beef jerky, instant oatmeal and rice, candy bars, and granola bars. These more easily digestible items are necessary for students and instructors to function in high Himalayan altitudes up to 18,000 feet.

NOLS AMAZON

NOLS Amazon is a new international NOLS base in the interior of Brazil on the southern limit of the Amazon Basin. This area, although remote, is still connected to the rapidly developing southeast Brazil and has many food options. The following list includes rations that are mostly unique to Brazil and a few that are found in NOLS's other international programs.

Black beans
Coffee
Condensed milk in cans (used to make the Brazilian desert brigadeiro)
Curau (hot sweet cornmeal cereal)
Dried Mushrooms

Dried tropical fruit (mango, papaya, guava, caqui, banana)
Farofa (manioc/yucca grain)
Goiaba (guava paste)
Maté
Miso
Pão de Queijo (manioc/yucca and cheese flour)
Salty Banana Chips
Soy products

NOLS also has bases in Baja, Mexico; Australia; and New Zealand. For rations information, please contact 1-800-710-NOLS.

THE NOLS RATIONING SYSTEM

Each year, approximately ten thousand students spend between fourteen and one hundred thirty-five days in the backcountry on NOLS courses. How does NOLS plan meals for so many people over such long periods? Each course is divided into cook groups of two to four individuals, and each cook group is given a wide selection of bulk foods and spices. They decide what to cook with the help of *NOLS Cookery*, as well as other knowledgeable peers or instructors. There are no set menus. Students learn how to cook in the field through experience.

We call this method NOLS bulk rationing and have found that it works well for our multiweek expeditions. Smaller groups going out for shorter lengths of time—five days or less—might want to consider menu planning instead (see *NOLS Backcountry Cooking: Creative Menu Planning for Short Trips*). With menu planning, all meals are determined in advance, and the food is bought accordingly.

► **Repackage food from the grocery store into large, zipper-lock bags to minimize packaging and to make sure foods are sealed well. Write meal preparation instructions in permanent marker on the plastic bags that hold the food.**

Successful ration planning takes both effort and experience, and it can be challenging and time-consuming. Critical factors to consider when planning for an expedition are the availability, versatility, cost, and palatability of desired foods. Happy campers must be well fed and hydrated. Plan for as much variety as possible, ask your trip members for their input, and organize most of the food ahead of time to ensure ease of preparation once in the field.

Factors to consider when ration planning:

Group size
Duration of trip
Purpose of trip
Exertion level
Weather
Altitude
Individual appetites
Food preferences within the group
Nutritional balance
Expense and availability
Spoilage and ease of packaging
Weight
Possible dietary limitations of group members

The first step in planning food for an expedition using the NOLS bulk rationing method is to calculate the total amount of food that will be needed during the trip. To do this, determine how many pounds of food per person per day (ppppd) you expect to use. (Charts and worksheets are included in this appendix to help you determine this figure.) Once you have figured out the total poundage, break it down into different food groups to get specific amounts. Make note of the food preferences and allergies within your group, and avoid letting your personal likes and dislikes influence your choices. Variety is important and will help keep up morale.

BULK RATION PLANNING STEPS

Step 1: *Determine the amount of food in pounds per person per day (ppppd), using the following guidelines:*

1.5 ppppd is appropriate for hot days and warm nights. This amount works well when base camping (camping in one location for the duration of the trip) and is good for short trips (three to five days) when fresh veggies, canned goods, and/or fresh fish supplement the ration. An excellent amount for trips with children and for leisure days, 1.5 pounds equates to roughly 2,500 to 3,000 calories per person per day.

1.75 to 2 ppppd works well when you expect warm or cool days and nights or when hiking with full packs. If you are planning a long trip of more than seven to ten days, you might want to plan on 2 ppppd for later in the ration period, since appetites usually kick in after a few days in the mountains. For moderate to active workdays, 1.75 to 2 pounds is ideal and gives you roughly 3,000 to 3,500 calories per person.

2 to 2.25 ppppd is good for hiking or skiing with full packs during the cool days and cold nights of early spring, late fall, or winter. If you are planning a long trip of more than seven to ten days, you might want to plan on 2.25 ppppd for later in the ration period. Two to 2.25 pounds per day is ideal for heavy workdays and cold temperatures. It gives you roughly 3,500 to 4,500 calories per person per day.

2.5 ppppd is good for cold days and extremely cold nights, such as in midwinter, when you are skiing with full packs or sleds in mountain environments. Used for extremely strenuous workdays and very cold temperatures, 2.5 pounds gives you roughly 4,000 to 5,000 calories per person per day.

Step 2: *Figure the total amount of food needed for the trip.* The formula is: Number of people multiplied by number of days multiplied by ppppd. For example, for four people on an eight-day trip at 1.75 ppppd, the total amount of food needed would equal 56 pounds.

Step 3: *Break the total poundage into food groups.* The following chart lists the breakdown of the poundage of different foods per person per day. Added together, these numbers (known as category multipliers) should equal the pounds per person per day selected in step 1. They have proved effective in planning NOLS rations for many years.

Category Multipliers

Food Category	*1.5 ppppd*	*1.75 ppppd*	*2 ppppd*	*2.25 ppppd*	*2.5 ppppd*
Breakfast	.24	.28	.33	.35	.38
Dinner	.27	.32	.35	.37	.40
Cheese	.19	.22	.24	.26	.28
Trail foods	.32	.35	.37	.45	.49
Flour and baking*	.11	.13	.16	.09	.10
Sugar and fruit drinks	.10	.12	.14	.15	.18
Soups, bases, desserts	.06	.09	.13	.15	.19
Milk, eggs, margarine, cocoa	.21	.24	.28	.31	.33
Meats and substitutes**	0	0	0	.12	.15

*The need for baking ingredients is lower in winter conditions, when only quick pan baking is feasible.

**High-fat and high-preservative meats are added in winter to meet higher fuel needs.

Step 4: *Calculate the total pounds of each food category needed for the trip.* Using the example from step 2 of four people on an eight-day trip at 1.75 ppppd and the category multipliers from the table in step 3, the calculations would be as follows:

Food Category	*Calculation*	*Rounded*
Trail foods	.35 × 4 × 8 = 11.2 lbs.	11 lbs.
Dinner	.32 × 4 × 8 = 10.24 lbs.	10.5 lbs.
Breakfast	.28 × 4 × 8 = 8.96 lbs.	9 lbs.

Milk, eggs, margarine, cocoa	.24 × 4 × 8 = 7.68 lbs.	7.5 lbs.
Cheese	.22 × 4 × 8 = 7.04 lbs.	7 lbs.
Flour and baking	.13 × 4 × 8 = 4.16 lbs.	4 lbs.
Sugar and fruit drinks	.12 × 4 × 8 = 3.84 lbs.	4 lbs.
Soups, bases, desserts	.09 × 4 × 8 = 2.88 lbs.	3 lbs.
Meats and substitutes	NOLS only uses in 2.25–2.5 lb. rations	
	Total pounds: 56 lbs.	

Step 5: *Round the numbers up or down within categories (see the last column of the table in step 4) and make substitutions, depending on individual preferences.* For instance, if you don't want to bake, you can take that poundage (approximately four pounds in the example) and add it to another category such as breakfast or dinner. If you don't eat cheese, you can take some of that cheese weight (approximately seven pounds in this example) and add it to the trail food category, where you can replace it with nuts and/or nut butters (sesame, peanut, tahini, or almond). The important thing to remember is to make exchanges with similar types of foods to maintain the balance among carbohydrates, proteins, and fats. If you make changes, the adjusted totals should still equal the amount determined in step 2.

The following worksheet can be used to plan your own ration.

RATION PLANNING WORKSHEET

If you have already chosen your pounds per person per day (ppppd), you are ready to fill in the worksheet.

Multiply the number of days times the number of people times the ppppd to find the total weight for the chosen ration period.

________ ×	________ ×	________ =	________
(days)	(people)	(ppppd)	(total weight)

Break down total weight into food categories (see step 3 in text).

Category	***No. of People***	×	***No. of Days***	×	***Category Multiplier***	=	***Total lbs. for Category***
Breakfast	________	×	________	×	________	=	________
Dinner	________	×	________	×	________	=	________
Cheese	________	×	________	×	________	=	________
Trail foods	________	×	________	×	________	=	________
Flour and baking	________	×	________	×	________	=	________
Sugar and fruit drinks	________	×	________	×	________	=	________
Soups, bases, desserts	________	×	________	×	________	=	________
Milk, eggs, margarine, cocoa	________	×	________	×	________	=	________
Meats and substitutes	________	×	________	×	________	=	________
					Total weight	=	________

Example (Trail foods, 1.5 ppppd): 4 people × 8 days × .35 ppppd = 11 total lbs.

List specific foods that you would like to take under each category listed below. You have generated these category totals in the formulas above.

Breakfast Item/lbs.	***Dinner Item/lbs.***	***Cheese Item/lbs.***	***Trail Foods Item/lbs.***	***Flour and Baking Item/lbs.***
________	________	________	________	________
________	________	________	________	________
________	________	________	________	________
________	________	________	________	________
________	________	________	________	________
________	________	________	________	________
Total lbs. _____	Total lbs. _____	Total lbs. _____	Total lbs. _____	Total lbs. _____

Sugar and Fruit Drinks Item/lbs.	***Soups, Bases, Desserts Item/lbs.***	***Milk, Eggs, Margarine, Cocoa Item/lbs.***	***Meats and Substitutes Item/lbs.***
________	________	________	________
________	________	________	________
________	________	________	________
________	________	________	________
________	________	________	________
________	________	________	________
Total lbs. _____	Total lbs. _____	Total lbs. _____	Total lbs. _____

At NOLS, we issue spice kits, tea bags, base packs, canned goods, fresh vegetables, toilet paper, matches, and soap (liquid or bar), in addition to the total weight planned for each ration. Make sure you include your choice of these items for your personal trips.

APPENDIX D

CALCULATE ENERGY (CALORIE) NEEDS

It is not necessary for most backcountry travelers to calculate their exact energy needs (nor is it possible to make exact calculations), but a rough estimate is a good idea for menu planning. Using the equations below, you can estimate a mellow rest day and a long, strenuous day in the field to plan a range of calories to meet your overall backcountry nutrition needs.

1. **Divide your body weight in pounds by 2.2 to get your weight in kilograms (kg). Then use the equation in the table for your age to calculate your Resting Energy Expenditure (REE).**

   Example:
   150 lbs. ÷ 2.2 = 68 kg
   18-year-old male: (15.3 × 68) + 679
   1,040 + 679 = 1,719 calories/day

Estimation of the Daily Resting Energy Expenditure (REE)[1]

Age (years)	*Equation*
Males	
10 to 17	(17.5 × body weight*) + 651
18 to 29	(15.3 × body weight) + 679
30 to 60	(11.6 × body weight) + 879

Estimation of the Daily Resting Energy Expenditure (REE)[1] (continued)	
Females	
10 to 17	(12.2 × body weight*) + 746
18 to 29	(14.7 × body weight) + 496
30 to 60	(8.7 × body weight) + 829

*Weight in kilograms (kg = pounds divided by 2.2; e.g., 150 lbs. ÷ 2.2 = 68 kg)

[1]REE does not include calories needed for physical activity—this is the baseline of calories used for basic functions.

2. **To calculate your Total Daily Energy Expenditure (TDEE) you will estimate the number of hours each day devoted to various activities, including rest and sleep. The multiples of Resting Energy Expenditure (REE) in the table below are multiplied by the number of hours for each activity and must total 24 hours.**

Physical Activity Factors	
Activity	***Multiple of REE***
Resting While at rest—sleeping, reading, etc.	**1.0**
Very light Sitting and standing activities—playing cards, writing, cooking, etc.	**1.5**
Light Activities that compare to walking at a leisurely pace—fishing from shore or boat, foraging for wild edibles, walking around camp (without a pack), etc.	**2.5**
Moderate Walking roughly 3.5 to 4 mph (with a light day pack or no pack), etc.	**5.0**
Heavy Walking or hiking faster, uphill (with or without a pack), running, or chopping firewood	**7.0**

Example: Using the 18-year-old male from above (REE = 1,719 calories/day) during a day in the backcountry that includes a mix of activities:

Resting or sleeping	9 hours × 1	= 9
Very light activity	4 hours × 1.5	= 6
Light Activity	3 hours × 2.5	= 7.5
Moderate activity	2 hours × 5.0	= 10
Heavy Activity	6 hours × 7.0	= 42
Totals	**24 hours**	**74.5**

Average physical activity quotient = 74.5 ÷ 24 = 3.10

TDEE = 3.10 x 1,719 = 5,329 calories per day

Based on our sample day, this 18-year-old backpacker will need approximately 5,329 calories for the day to meet his nutritional needs. There are other factors not accounted for here, such as weather or extreme environmental conditions that could increase these needs. There are also variables such as the exact weight of his pack that could potentially decrease his calorie needs. The idea is to get an estimate. Ideally, you can determine a range of calories based on calculations of a lightly active and a more strenuous day.

APPENDIX E

1999 NOLS ROCKY MOUNTAIN NUTRITION STUDY

In August 1999, Claudia Pearson, rations manager at NOLS Rocky Mountain, spearheaded a study of the standard summer rations for NOLS to determine nutritional adequacy and assess the overall nutritional quality of the rations. Seven sample field rations were analyzed using a computerized nutritional analysis program (ESHA—Food Processor version 6.0, ESHA Research, Salem, OR 1996). The ESHA database was expanded to include items specific to NOLS rations based on food labels and information from manufacturers. Unfortunately, manufacturers are not required to provide extensive micronutrient information (vitamins and minerals). Due to the lack of nutrition information regarding the full spectrum of micronutrients, this study focused on the macronutrients protein, carbohydrate, and fat.

The results of this study showed an adequate amount of total carbohydrates and a fiber content that met or exceeded the recommended 11.5 grams per 1,000 calories. The total amount of calories in the rations studied averaged 3,200 per day. The amount of fat was slightly higher than the recommended 30 percent of total calories as shown in the following table, and approximately 6 percent higher than the recommendations of many sports nutritionists (fat content 25 percent of total calories). The protein amounts averaged 92 grams per day and 11 percent of total calories. This amount is adequate for the active one-hundred-twenty-five-pound individual, but it is a bit low for everyone else. The protein recommendations for endurance athletes are in the 1 to 1.6 grams per kilogram per day range.

Results of 1999 NOLS Nutrition Study

Averages based on sample of rations (n = 7)

Nutrient Studied	*Average amount (g)*	*Average % of total calories*	*Recommended % of total calories**
Carbohydrate	480.56	58.79	50–75
Protein	92.49	11.29	10–15
Fat	113.39	31.31	≤ 30

*World Health Organization, 1995.

There are a few key points to consider when reviewing these results. The analysis was completed using course bag sheets from seven different samples of NOLS summer field rations. The total number of pounds of items issued was entered into the nutrition analysis computer program and then divided by the number of days and the number of people for each course.

The obvious limitations to this method of analysis are that the results are based on even distribution and complete consumption of the rations. It is common knowledge that some individuals eat more than others do, evacuations occur and allow for different distribution of foods among students remaining in the field, and some foods are returned at the completion of the course. This means that some NOLS people may be getting adequate nutrients while others may not, depending upon the choices made in the field with regard to the consumption of rations issued. The analysis also did not consider the addition of fresh produce, canned goods, fresh fish, or special items that may be issued or brought from home to supplement basic rations. Despite these limitations, this study was a good baseline assessment of the macronutrients available in the standard Rocky Mountain field rations for NOLS students and instructors.

The results of this study are consistent with concerns voiced by a few NOLS instructors, as well as some of the student course evaluations regarding the amount of protein available in the NOLS rations. The degree to which the NOLS rations may be low in protein amounts to 0 to 30 grams less than the recommendation, depending upon the size of the individual and the food choices the individual makes in the field. This is about 3 percent less than the desired proportion of total calories, assuming highly active NOLS folk need to be at the upper end of the recommendations for protein (15 percent of total calories). This level of protein intake, however, is not likely to cause any major symptoms of protein deficiency.

Based upon instructor and student comments, most NOLS people were satisfied with the rations and reported no feelings of nutrient deficits. There were a few instructors that reported feeling "run down" after multiple courses and attributed this feeling to inadequate protein. This is obviously a difficult phenomenon to assess properly without conducting nitrogen balance studies, particularly since there are several factors that contribute to fatigue and compromised immune function. In fact, both fatigue and immune dysfunction can be caused by insufficient carbohydrate to keep blood sugar levels steady and glycogen stores full. Other factors that affect both energy levels and immune function include dehydration, low iron levels, and inadequate calorie intake over time in the field.

The bottom line is that dietary protein *may or may not* be a factor of fatigue. Given the influence instructors have on NOLS students, it is especially important for them to stay open when assessing the possible causes of fatigue. Even though the NOLS rations provide ample carbohydrates, it is possible for students to fill up on the cheese and not take in adequate carbohydrates to fuel working muscles, and it is even more probable that students are not properly hydrated at all times. As was discussed in the water chapter of this book, the fluid requirements on a NOLS course are substantially higher than any out-of-the-field physical activity. Living outdoors, often at higher altitudes, involves increased physical activity beyond hiking, climbing, or skiing; just going from the kiva to the kitchen or bathroom may be an uphill hike. Then there is the added challenge of hot or cold environments that increase fluid needs.

Some instructors that have pinpointed inadequate protein intake as the likely culprit for fatigue choose to pack in supplemental protein sources in the form of tinned meats or fish, jerky, sausage, and energy bars that contain protein. For larger individuals who need 130 grams of protein per day, these are probably good options. This is also important for instructors who depend upon the NOLS rations to sustain their own health and extensive physical activity for a big chunk of the year in order to keep meals interesting. One note regarding the energy bars is, yes, they contain protein, but they also provide carbohydrates and a number of potentially significant vitamins and minerals that may contribute to the feeling of well-being associated with this supplement choice. Again, it is not a given that the protein portion of these bars is actually making the difference in energy levels or immune function.

APPENDIX F SAMPLE ANALYSES OF BACKCOUNTRY FIELD MENUS

Estimating your calorie and other nutrient needs is a good step towards making sure you are well nourished in the backcountry, but knowing what a certain range of calories looks like when applied to real food is a practical next step. If you are eating a variety of foods throughout the day and drinking plenty of water and you are feeling healthy, happy and energetic, then you are probably getting what you need. Unfortunately, as several chapters in this book point out, there are situations in the backcountry when your appetite may be suppressed (high-altitude travel, strenuous exercise, heat, and humidity), and you may need to eat despite a lack of hunger. The knowledge of a "typical day in the field" may help you to eat enough on the days when your body isn't prompting you properly.

In the frontcountry it is easy to get more calories than we need. But, during extended trips in the backcountry where we must carry our provisions and prepare all of our meals, it can be more difficult to get enough calories. This appendix provides three different sample backcountry days ranging from 2,500 to 4,000 calories.

The first example is a NOLS female eating roughly 2,500 calories for the day. The second example is a male Appalachian Trail hiker based on one of the nutrition surveys described in appendix G. The third sample day uses the 3,000-calorie day introduced in the energy chapter and compares it to the needs of a very active backcountry female and male. The day's intake ends up a bit high for the female and low for the male. There is a discussion about how to easily adjust the menu to suit the needs of each backcountry adventurer and an analysis of the modified backcountry male's day in the field to show what roughly 4,000 calories looks like when applied to backcountry foods.

It is important to keep in mind that all of these recommendations are estimates. Real life backcountry situations may require more or fewer calories and other nutrients. The computer program used to analyze these menus (ESHA Food Processor for Windows version 7.9, ESHA Research, Salem, OR 2002)

Sample Backcountry Menu for NOLS Student—2,500-calorie Day in the Field

Food	*Amount*	*Calories*
Breakfast		
NOLS pancake mix	1 cup mix (122 g)	422
Margarine	2 Tbs.	203
Peanut butter	3 Tbs.	285
Hot cider	1 packet	83
(From this breakfast, 2 mini pancakes + 1 Tbs. peanut butter were taken to eat as a trail snack—roughly 250 calories of this breakfast.)		
On the Trail (throughout the day)		
Chocolate covered raisins	1/2 cup	371
High-fiber crackers	4	59
Hummus (from mix)	3 Tbs.	90
Fruit and oatmeal bar	1	136
NOLS Fiesta snack mix	2 oz.	243
Back at Camp		
Bow tie pasta	3 oz. (1 cup+)	309
Tomato powder	2 Tbs.	42
Bullion cube	1 cube	11
Mozzarella cheese	3 cubes (1″ ea)	238
Hot cocoa	1 packet	70
Totals		**2,562 calories**

uses standard recommendations based on age, height, weight, and a "very active" activity level (defined as "full-time athlete"). The protein recommendations are based on a percentage of total calories rather than the .6 to .9 gram per pound of body weight calculation introduced in the protein chapter for endurance athletes. This means the protein needs may be higher than the amount shown in the bar graph analyses. The analysis does give the number of grams of protein for each of the sample days so you can use this information to compare to your own calculations for protein.

This menu is a sample day in the field for a thirty-year-old very active NOLS female. The nutrition profile that follows uses standard recommendations based on her age (30), height (5′3″), weight (125 lbs.) and activity level (very active—characterized as full-time athletes). The protein recommendations are based on a percentage of total calories rather than the .6 to .9 grams per pound of body weight calculation introduced in the protein chapter for endurance athletes. Using the adjusted protein recommendations this female may actually be below her protein needs on this day. If this were a day early in her backcountry journey when she is still building muscle and adjusting to the increased demands of backcountry travel and living, she may want to include some additional protein at meals or snacks. However, she is taking in more than the recommended amount for basic functions for a very active lifestyle.

Nutrition Profile Very Active NOLS Female

Female	30 yrs	5 ft 3 in	125 lbs	Very Active	BMI: 22.14

Basic Components		
Calories	2513.49	
Calories from Fat	754.05	
Calories from Saturated Fat	226.21	
Protein	45.36	g
Carbohydrates	364.46	g
Dietary Fiber	28.91	g
Fat - Total	83.78	g
Saturated Fat	25.13	g
Mono Fat	30.72	g
Poly Fat	27.93	g
Cholesterol	300.00	mg

Vitamins		
Vitamin A IU	3500.00	IU
Vitamin A RAE	700.00	RAE
Vitamin A RE	700.00	RE
Thiamin-B1	1.10	mg
Riboflavin-B2	1.10	mg
Niacin-B3	14.00	mg
Niacin Equiv.	14.00	mg
Vitamin-B6	1.30	mg
Vitamin-B12	2.40	mcg
Biotin	30.00	mcg
Vitamin C	75.00	mg
Vitamin D IU	200.00	IU
Vitamin D mcg	5.00	mcg
Vit E Alpha-Tocopherol	15.00	AToco
Vit E-Alpha Equiv.	15.00	mg
Folate	400.00	mcg
Folate DFE	400.00	DFE
Vitamin K	90.00	mcg
Pantothenic Acid	5.00	mg

Minerals		
Calcium	1000.00	mg
Chromium	25.00	mcg
Copper	0.90	mg
Fluoride	3.00	mg
Iodine	150.00	mcg
Iron	18.00	mg
Magnesium	310.00	mg
Manganese	1.80	mg
Molybdenum	45.00	mcg
Phosphorus	700.00	mg
Potassium	3500.00	mg
Selenium	55.00	mcg
Sodium	2400.00	mg
Zinc	8.00	mg

Other		
Choline	425.00	mg

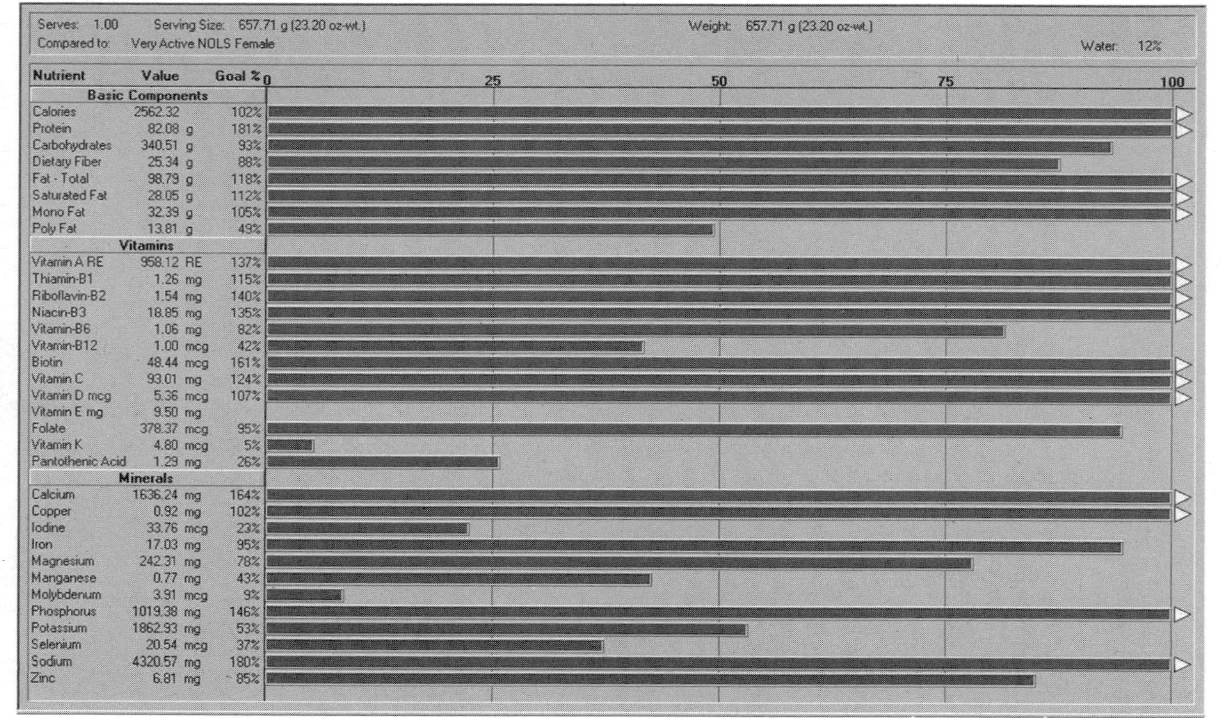

Serves: 1.00 Serving Size: 657.71 g (23.20 oz-wt.) Weight: 657.71 g (23.20 oz-wt.) Water: 12%
Compared to: Very Active NOLS Female

Nutrient	Value	Goal %
Basic Components		
Calories	2562.32	102%
Protein	82.08 g	181%
Carbohydrates	340.51 g	93%
Dietary Fiber	25.34 g	88%
Fat - Total	98.79 g	118%
Saturated Fat	28.05 g	112%
Mono Fat	32.39 g	105%
Poly Fat	13.81 g	49%
Vitamins		
Vitamin A RE	958.12 RE	137%
Thiamin-B1	1.26 mg	115%
Riboflavin-B2	1.54 mg	140%
Niacin-B3	18.85 mg	135%
Vitamin-B6	1.06 mg	82%
Vitamin-B12	1.00 mcg	42%
Biotin	48.44 mcg	161%
Vitamin C	93.01 mg	124%
Vitamin D mcg	5.36 mcg	107%
Vitamin E mg	9.50 mg	
Folate	378.37 mcg	95%
Vitamin K	4.80 mcg	5%
Pantothenic Acid	1.29 mg	26%
Minerals		
Calcium	1636.24 mg	164%
Copper	0.92 mg	102%
Iodine	33.76 mcg	23%
Iron	17.03 mg	95%
Magnesium	242.31 mg	78%
Manganese	0.77 mg	43%
Molybdenum	3.91 mcg	9%
Phosphorus	1019.38 mg	146%
Potassium	1862.93 mg	53%
Selenium	20.54 mcg	37%
Sodium	4320.57 mg	180%
Zinc	6.81 mg	85%

As you can see from this nutrient analysis, our NOLS student is meeting her needs for all of the basic nutrients (with the possible exception of protein, depending on how you estimate it). Ideally if she varies her intake throughout her trip, she will take in more of the nutrients that came in below the 75 percent mark on other days. If you are interested in food sources to increase some of these nutrients (manganese, selenium, vitamins E, B12, and pantothenic acid), you can refer to the vitamin and mineral tables in chapter 6.

Sample Appalachian Trail Hiker 3,000-Calorie Day

23-year-old male, 6′1″, 170 lbs. (77 kg)
Estimate for very active day (approximately 6 hours moderate hiking with a pack) somewhere between 3,057 and 3,843 calories.

Food	*Amount*	*Calories*
Breakfast		
Frosted blueberry Pop-Tarts	2	407
Hot cocoa, Nestle	1 packet	112
On the Trail (throughout the day)		
Snickers candy bar	1 (2 oz.)	272
Kool-Aid drink mix, orange	60 grams (3 Tbs. mix)	212
Dry roasted peanuts	42 grams (1.5 oz. pkg.)	246
Beef jerky	3 pieces	244
Cheese crackers with peanut butter filling	6 crackers	202
Back at Camp		
Mountain House Mexican Rice and Chicken Dinner	1 whole pkg. (2 svgs.)	640
Cheddar cheese	4 oz.	457
Totals		**3,061 calories**

Nutrition Profile AT male 23 yo hiker

Male | 23 yrs | 6 ft 1 in | 170 lbs | Very Active | BMI: 22.43

Basic Components		
Calories	3843.79	
Calories from Fat	1153.17	
Calories from Saturated Fat	345.96	
Protein	61.69	g
Carbohydrates	557.35	g
Dietary Fiber	44.20	g
Fat - Total	128.13	g
Saturated Fat	38.44	g
Mono Fat	46.98	g
Poly Fat	42.71	g
Cholesterol	300.00	mg

Vitamins		
Vitamin A IU	4500.00	IU
Vitamin A RAE	900.00	RAE
Vitamin A RE	900.00	RE
Thiamin-B1	1.20	mg
Riboflavin-B2	1.30	mg
Niacin-B3	16.00	mg
Niacin Equiv.	16.00	mg
Vitamin-B6	1.30	mg
Vitamin-B12	2.40	mcg
Biotin	30.00	mcg
Vitamin C	90.00	mg
Vitamin D IU	200.00	IU
Vitamin D mcg	5.00	mcg
Vit E Alpha-Tocopherol	15.00	AToco
Vit E-Alpha Equiv.	15.00	mg
Folate	400.00	mcg
Folate DFE	400.00	DFE
Vitamin K	120.00	mcg
Pantothenic Acid	5.00	mg

Minerals		
Calcium	1000.00	mg
Chromium	35.00	mcg
Copper	0.90	mg
Fluoride	4.00	mg
Iodine	150.00	mcg
Iron	8.00	mg
Magnesium	400.00	mg
Manganese	2.30	mg
Molybdenum	45.00	mcg
Phosphorus	700.00	mg
Potassium	3500.00	mg
Selenium	55.00	mcg
Sodium	2400.00	mg
Zinc	11.00	mg

Other		
Choline	550.00	mg

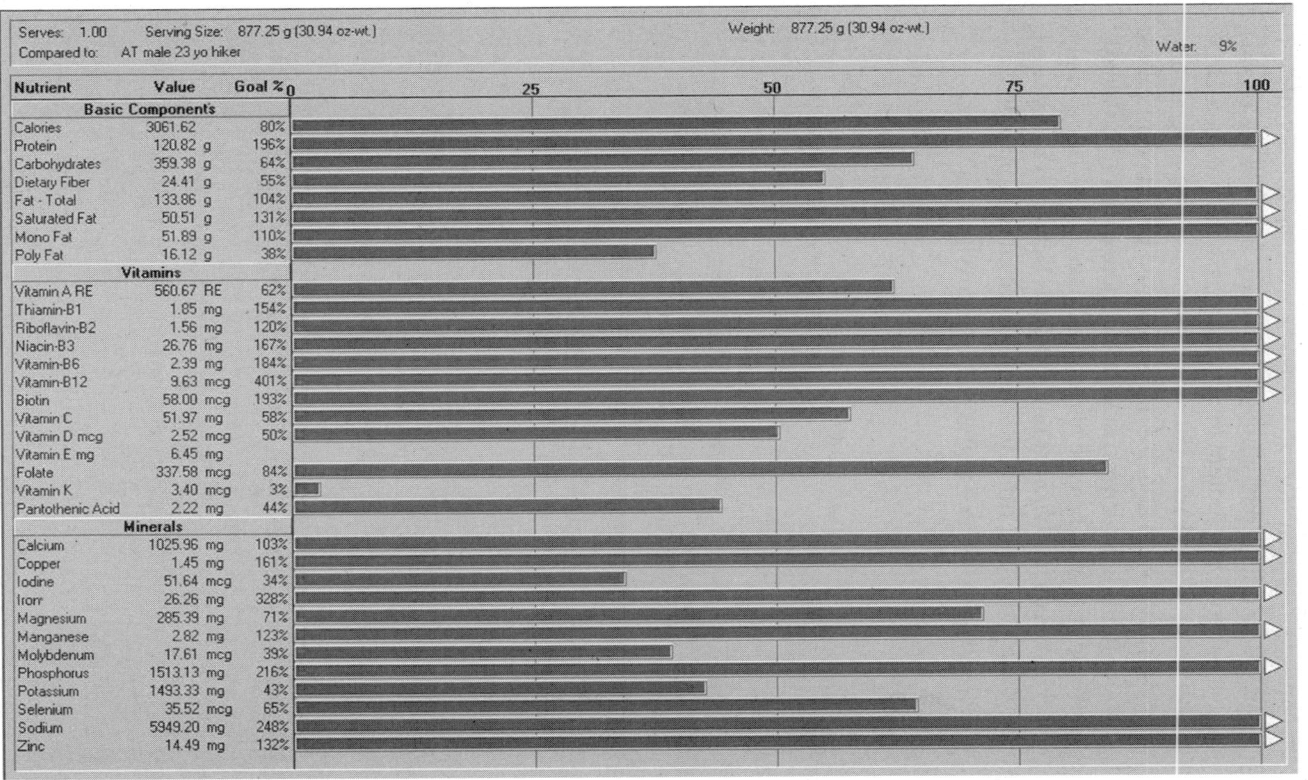

Serves: 1.00 Serving Size: 877.25 g (30.94 oz-wt.) Weight: 877.25 g (30.94 oz-wt.) Water: 9%

Compared to: AT male 23 yo hiker

Nutrient	Value	Goal %
Basic Components		
Calories	3061.62	80%
Protein	120.82 g	196%
Carbohydrates	359.38 g	64%
Dietary Fiber	24.41 g	55%
Fat - Total	133.86 g	104%
Saturated Fat	50.51 g	131%
Mono Fat	51.89 g	110%
Poly Fat	16.12 g	38%
Vitamins		
Vitamin A RE	560.67 RE	62%
Thiamin-B1	1.85 mg	154%
Riboflavin-B2	1.56 mg	120%
Niacin-B3	26.76 mg	167%
Vitamin-B6	2.39 mg	184%
Vitamin-B12	9.63 mcg	401%
Biotin	58.00 mcg	193%
Vitamin C	51.97 mg	58%
Vitamin D mcg	2.52 mcg	50%
Vitamin E mg	6.45 mg	
Folate	337.58 mcg	84%
Vitamin K	3.40 mcg	3%
Pantothenic Acid	2.22 mg	44%
Minerals		
Calcium	1025.96 mg	103%
Copper	1.45 mg	161%
Iodine	51.64 mcg	34%
Iron	26.26 mg	328%
Magnesium	285.39 mg	71%
Manganese	2.82 mg	123%
Molybdenum	17.61 mcg	39%
Phosphorus	1513.13 mg	216%
Potassium	1493.33 mg	43%
Selenium	35.52 mcg	65%
Sodium	5949.20 mg	248%
Zinc	14.49 mg	132%

As you can see from the nutrient analysis of our male AT hiker, his calorie, carbohydrate, and dietary fiber intakes on this day are all low. His sodium intake was very high, not necessarily a bad thing in the backcountry, but his potassium, magnesium, and vitamin E were also low. If he increased his intake of carbohydrate foods with some snacks and a more balanced breakfast, he would not only increase his calorie intake but he could easily meet his needs for the other nutrients he is lacking. If he replaced the Kool-Aid with a drink mix that is fortified with vitamin C he could bring up the level of this vitamin as well.

A rough estimate of a highly active backcountry day is often 3,000 calories. This menu appears in chapter 2 as an illustration of what 3,000 calories looks like when applied to some common backcountry foods. Following the menu you will see the nutrition profiles for a very active backcountry female and male. You will then find a nutrient analysis that compares this sample menu to each of these backcountry travelers' needs.

Sample 3,000-Calorie Day Backcountry Menu (shown in chapter 2)

Food	*Amount*	*Calories*
Breakfast		
Instant oatmeal	2 packets	209
Raisins	1/4 cup	109
Walnut halves	1/4 cup	164
Powdered milk, for cereal and extra for cocoa	1/2 cup	122
Hot cocoa	1 packet	70
On the Trail (throughout the day)		
Yogurt-covered peanuts	1/2 cup	460
Bagel, plain	one, 3″	157
Cheddar cheese, sharp	2 oz.	240
Fig bar cookies	4	223
Soy nuts, salted	1 oz. (1/3 cup)	120
Clif Bar or choc. brownie	1	236
Tang, orange	2 tbs	92
Back at Camp		
Macaroni and cheese	2 cups	820
Sun-dried tomatoes	4 pieces	21
Herbal tea	12 oz.	3
Hot cocoa	1 packet	70
Totals		**3,115 calories**

Profile for a very active backcountry female, twenty-five years of age, 5′4″, and, 125 lbs.

Nutrition Profile Backcountry Female

Female | 25 yrs | 5 ft 4 in | 125 lbs | Very Active | BMI: 21.46

Basic Components	
Calories	2519.19
Calories from Fat	755.73
Calories from Saturated Fat	226.71
Protein	45.36 g
Carbohydrates	365.28 g
Dietary Fiber	28.97 g
Fat - Total	83.97 g
Saturated Fat	25.19 g
Mono Fat	30.79 g
Poly Fat	27.99 g
Cholesterol	300.00 mg

Vitamins	
Vitamin A IU	3500.00 IU
Vitamin A RAE	700.00 RAE
Vitamin A RE	700.00 RE
Thiamin-B1	1.10 mg
Riboflavin-B2	1.10 mg
Niacin-B3	14.00 mg
Niacin Equiv.	14.00 mg
Vitamin-B6	1.30 mg
Vitamin-B12	2.40 mcg
Biotin	30.00 mcg
Vitamin C	75.00 mg
Vitamin D IU	200.00 IU
Vitamin D mcg	5.00 mcg
Vit E Alpha-Tocopherol	15.00 AToco
Vit E-Alpha Equiv.	15.00 mg
Folate	400.00 mcg
Folate DFE	400.00 DFE
Vitamin K	90.00 mcg
Pantothenic Acid	5.00 mg

Minerals	
Calcium	1000.00 mg
Chromium	25.00 mcg
Copper	0.90 mg
Fluoride	3.00 mg
Iodine	150.00 mcg
Iron	18.00 mg
Magnesium	310.00 mg
Manganese	1.80 mg
Molybdenum	45.00 mcg
Phosphorus	700.00 mg
Potassium	3500.00 mg
Selenium	55.00 mcg
Sodium	2400.00 mg
Zinc	8.00 mg

Other	
Choline	425.00 mg

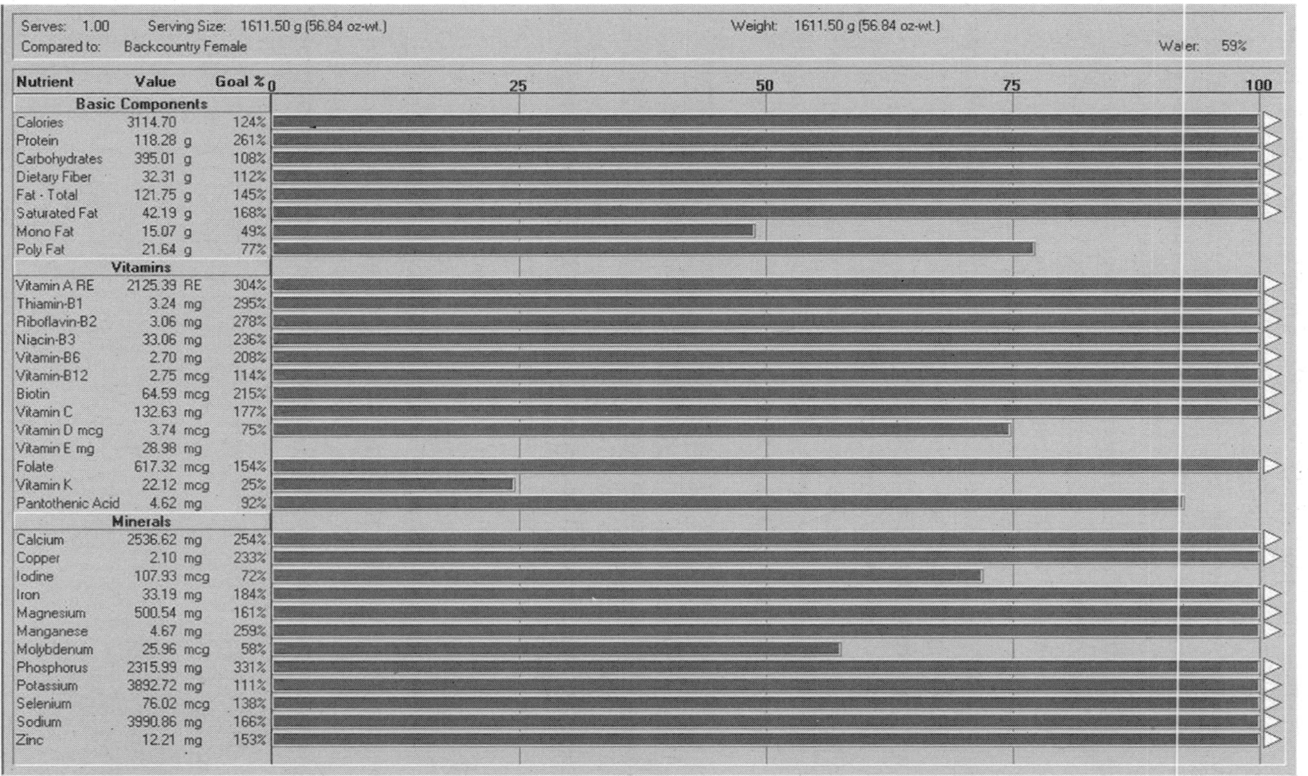

Serves: 1.00 Serving Size: 1611.50 g (56.84 oz-wt.) Weight: 1611.50 g (56.84 oz-wt.)
Compared to: Backcountry Female Water: 59%

Nutrient	Value	Goal %
Basic Components		
Calories	3114.70	124%
Protein	118.28 g	261%
Carbohydrates	395.01 g	108%
Dietary Fiber	32.31 g	112%
Fat - Total	121.75 g	145%
Saturated Fat	42.19 g	168%
Mono Fat	15.07 g	49%
Poly Fat	21.64 g	77%
Vitamins		
Vitamin A RE	2125.39 RE	304%
Thiamin-B1	3.24 mg	295%
Riboflavin-B2	3.06 mg	278%
Niacin-B3	33.06 mg	236%
Vitamin-B6	2.70 mg	208%
Vitamin-B12	2.75 mcg	114%
Biotin	64.59 mcg	215%
Vitamin C	132.63 mg	177%
Vitamin D mcg	3.74 mcg	75%
Vitamin E mg	28.98 mg	
Folate	617.32 mcg	154%
Vitamin K	22.12 mcg	25%
Pantothenic Acid	4.62 mg	92%
Minerals		
Calcium	2536.62 mg	254%
Copper	2.10 mg	233%
Iodine	107.93 mcg	72%
Iron	33.19 mg	184%
Magnesium	500.54 mg	161%
Manganese	4.67 mg	259%
Molybdenum	25.96 mcg	58%
Phosphorus	2315.99 mg	331%
Potassium	3892.72 mg	111%
Selenium	76.02 mcg	138%
Sodium	3990.86 mg	166%
Zinc	12.21 mg	153%

This analysis shows that the 3,000-calorie sample field menu is more than this backcountry female may need for a very active day. She has taken in roughly 500 calories more than she needs according to this estimate. This looks like a lot of extra calories, and in the frontcountry it is enough to gain 1 to 2 pounds in a week, if every day was over by 500 calories. In the backcountry, however, nutritional needs can vary dramatically from day to day. There are also many variables this program doesn't take into account when it analyzes her needs (environmental conditions, the exact amount of physical activity, pack weight, and individual metabolism). In most cases, taking in extra calories in the backcountry on one day will probably be balanced on other days. However, if we did want to readjust the calories to more accurately meet her estimated needs, substitutions can be made. Just three simple changes can put her into the desired range:

- Decrease the portion of macaroni and cheese at dinner from 2 cups to 1½ cups (205 fewer calories)
- Reduce the yogurt-covered peanuts to ¼ cup (instead of ½ cup) to save another 230 calories
- Take away either 1 ounce of cheese (120 fewer calories) or 2 fig cookies (110 fewer calories)

Next we have a very active backcountry male, twenty years of age, 6′0″, and 180 lbs.

As you will see, the 3,000-calorie menu is significantly less than the estimated needs for this backcountry male. He is approximately 900 calories below his target, low in both carbohydrates and fiber yet, surprisingly, he is within the range of protein recommendations using the .6 to .9 gram per pound of body weight (108 to 162 grams per day).

Nutrition Profile Backcountry Male

Male	20 yrs	6 ft 0 in	180 lbs	Very Active	BMI: 24.41

Basic Components	
Calories	4031.38
Calories from Fat	1209.42
Calories from Saturated Fat	362.79
Protein	65.32 g
Carbohydrates	584.55 g
Dietary Fiber	46.36 g
Fat - Total	134.38 g
Saturated Fat	40.31 g
Mono Fat	49.27 g
Poly Fat	44.79 g
Cholesterol	300.00 mg
Vitamins	
Vitamin A IU	4500.00 IU
Vitamin A RAE	900.00 RAE
Vitamin A RE	900.00 RE
Thiamin-B1	1.20 mg
Riboflavin-B2	1.30 mg
Niacin-B3	16.00 mg
Niacin Equiv.	16.00 mg
Vitamin-B6	1.30 mg
Vitamin-B12	2.40 mcg
Biotin	30.00 mcg
Vitamin C	90.00 mg
Vitamin D IU	200.00 IU
Vitamin D mcg	5.00 mcg
Vit E Alpha-Tocopherol	15.00 AToco
Vit E-Alpha Equiv.	15.00 mg
Folate	400.00 mcg
Folate DFE	400.00 DFE
Vitamin K	120.00 mcg
Pantothenic Acid	5.00 mg
Minerals	
Calcium	1000.00 mg
Chromium	35.00 mcg
Copper	0.90 mg
Fluoride	4.00 mg
Iodine	150.00 mcg
Iron	8.00 mg
Magnesium	400.00 mg
Manganese	2.30 mg
Molybdenum	45.00 mcg
Phosphorus	700.00 mg
Potassium	3500.00 mg
Selenium	55.00 mcg
Sodium	2400.00 mg
Zinc	11.00 mg
Other	
Choline	550.00 mg

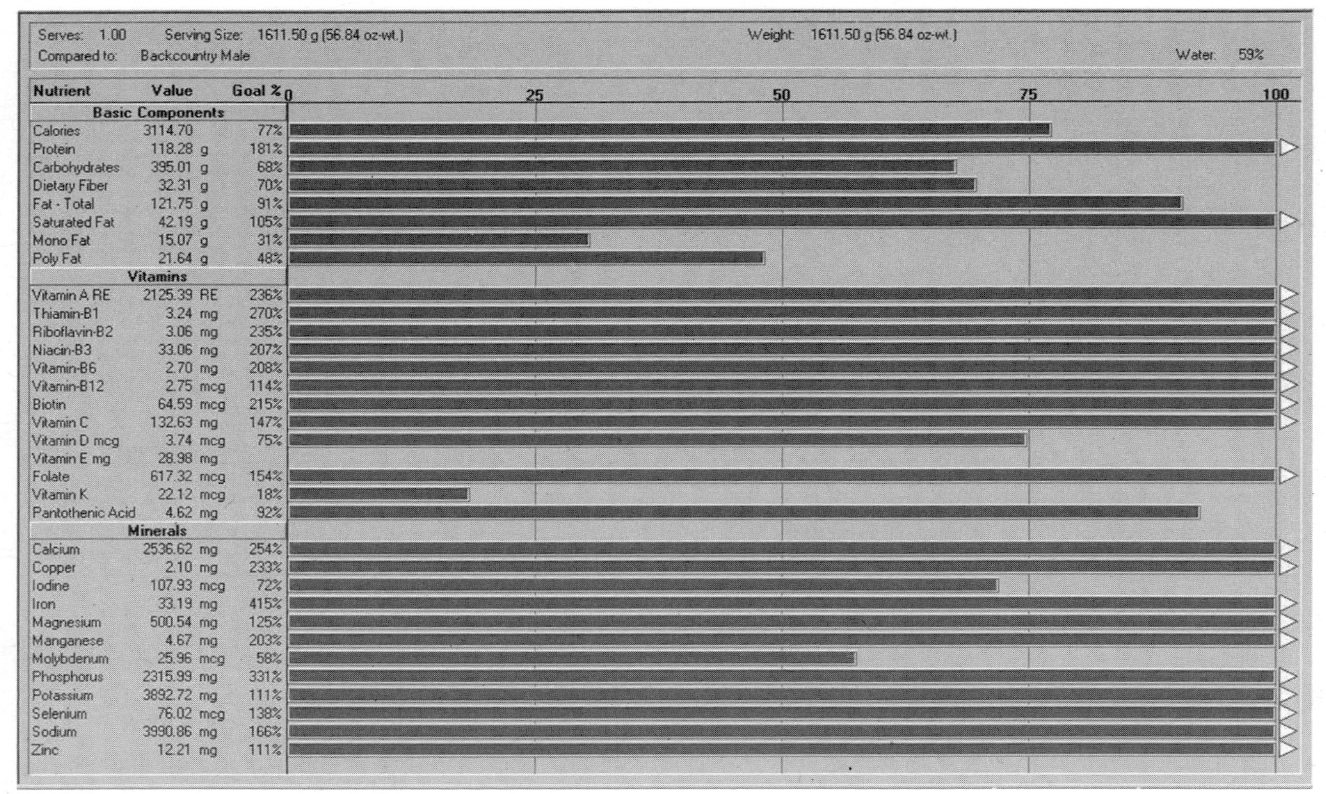

Serves: 1.00 Serving Size: 1611.50 g (56.84 oz-wt.) Weight: 1611.50 g (56.84 oz-wt.)
Compared to: Backcountry Male Water: 59%

Nutrient	Value	Goal %
Basic Components		
Calories	3114.70	77%
Protein	118.28 g	181%
Carbohydrates	395.01 g	68%
Dietary Fiber	32.31 g	70%
Fat - Total	121.75 g	91%
Saturated Fat	42.19 g	105%
Mono Fat	15.07 g	31%
Poly Fat	21.64 g	48%
Vitamins		
Vitamin A RE	2125.39 RE	236%
Thiamin-B1	3.24 mg	270%
Riboflavin-B2	3.06 mg	235%
Niacin-B3	33.06 mg	207%
Vitamin-B6	2.70 mg	208%
Vitamin-B12	2.75 mcg	114%
Biotin	64.59 mcg	215%
Vitamin C	132.63 mg	147%
Vitamin D mcg	3.74 mcg	75%
Vitamin E mg	28.98 mg	
Folate	617.32 mcg	154%
Vitamin K	22.12 mcg	18%
Pantothenic Acid	4.62 mg	92%
Minerals		
Calcium	2536.62 mg	254%
Copper	2.10 mg	233%
Iodine	107.93 mcg	72%
Iron	33.19 mg	415%
Magnesium	500.54 mg	125%
Manganese	4.67 mg	203%
Molybdenum	25.96 mcg	58%
Phosphorus	2315.99 mg	331%
Potassium	3892.72 mg	111%
Selenium	76.02 mcg	138%
Sodium	3990.86 mg	166%
Zinc	12.21 mg	111%

While a deficit of nearly 1,000 calories is a lot of food, modifying this menu to accommodate this backcountry male's needs is not as difficult as you may think. In fact, the modification actually went over the calorie needs by almost 200 calories:

3,000-Calorie Sample Field Menu Modified to Approximately 4,000 Calories

	Food	*Amount*	*Calories*
Breakfast			
	Instant oatmeal	2 packets	209
	Raisins	1/4 cup	109
	Walnut halves	1/4 cup	164
	Powdered milk (cereal and extra for cocoa)	1/2 cup	122
	Hot cocoa	1 packet	70
ADD:	Powdered milk	1/4 cup	60
	Raisins	1/4 cup	109
	Grape Nuts cereal	1/4 cup	208
On the Trail (throughout the day)			
	Yogurt-covered peanuts	1/2 cup	460
	Bagel, (plain)	one, 3″	157
ADD:	Peanut butter	2 Tbs.	190
	Honey	2 Tbs.	129
	Cheddar cheese, sharp	2 oz.	240
	Fig bar cookies	4	223
	Soy nuts, salted	1 oz. (1/3 cup)	120
ADD:	Soy nuts, salted	1 oz.	120
	Clif Bar or choc. brownie	1	236
	Tang, orange	2 Tbs.	92
ADD:	Tang, orange drink mix	2 Tbs.	92
Back at Camp			
	Macaroni and cheese	2 cups	820
ADD:	Macaroni and cheese	1/2 cup	205
	Sun-dried tomatoes	6 pieces	31
	Herbal tea	12 oz.	3
	Hot cocoa	1 packet	70
Total			**4,238 calories**

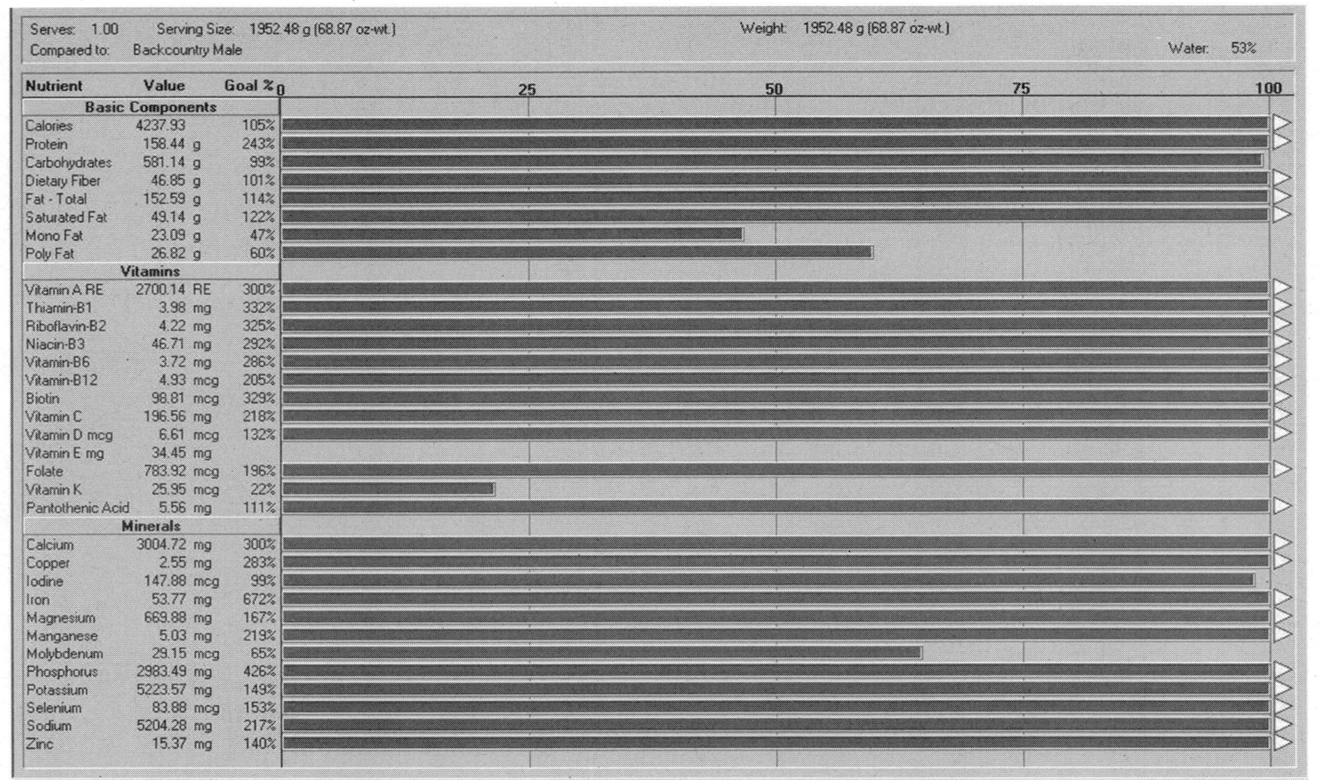

Nutrient	Value	Goal %
Basic Components		
Calories	4237.93	105%
Protein	158.44 g	243%
Carbohydrates	581.14 g	99%
Dietary Fiber	46.85 g	101%
Fat - Total	152.59 g	114%
Saturated Fat	49.14 g	122%
Mono Fat	23.09 g	47%
Poly Fat	26.82 g	60%
Vitamins		
Vitamin A RE	2700.14 RE	300%
Thiamin-B1	3.98 mg	332%
Riboflavin-B2	4.22 mg	325%
Niacin-B3	46.71 mg	292%
Vitamin-B6	3.72 mg	286%
Vitamin-B12	4.93 mcg	205%
Biotin	98.81 mcg	329%
Vitamin C	196.56 mg	218%
Vitamin D mcg	6.61 mcg	132%
Vitamin E mg	34.45 mg	
Folate	783.92 mcg	196%
Vitamin K	25.95 mcg	22%
Pantothenic Acid	5.56 mg	111%
Minerals		
Calcium	3004.72 mg	300%
Copper	2.55 mg	283%
Iodine	147.88 mcg	99%
Iron	53.77 mg	672%
Magnesium	669.88 mg	167%
Manganese	5.03 mg	219%
Molybdenum	29.15 mcg	65%
Phosphorus	2983.49 mg	426%
Potassium	5223.57 mg	149%
Selenium	83.88 mcg	153%
Sodium	5204.28 mg	217%
Zinc	15.37 mg	140%

Basically, the following changes made the difference:

- More food at breakfast (milk, raisins, and some grape nuts cereal stirred into the oatmeal)
- Larger portions of trail snacks (soy nuts or cheese) and drink mix
- A peanut butter and honey bagel for lunch on the trail
- A larger portion of macaroni and cheese at dinner (with some extra sun-dried tomatoes, more to keep it realistic in terms of increasing the portion than to add calories)

APPENDIX G APPALACHIAN TRAIL NUTRITION SURVEY

While co-presenting a workshop about various approaches to backcountry meal planning with Dr. Wayne Askew from the University of Utah at the Wilderness Medical Society's winter meeting in 2000, a discussion began among the participants regarding the lack of research about what the average person actually eats in the backcountry. After the session, Dr. George Wortley approached me about conducting a nutrition survey for Appalachian Trail (AT) hikers. Dr. Wortley has a medical practice in Virginia, located fairly close to two different trailheads that access the AT. So, he and I collaborated to write a brief survey and, during the summer and fall of 2000, Dr. Wortley collected data from 428 backcountry hikers.

Due to the demands of finishing my master's thesis, researching and writing the 2002 *NOLS Nutrition Field Guide*, and then establishing my nutrition counseling practice, the surveys have been tucked away in a box until this writing. Although we have not formally analyzed the data collected for this project, I wanted at least to present in this book some of the findings and anecdotes from the surveys. I am very grateful for the many hikers who took the time to complete these surveys and for the time Dr. Wortley devoted to administering and collecting them. Even though this data was collected several years ago, based upon my experience teaching backcountry nutrition classes more recently, the responses appear to remain representative of many hikers who spend extended time in the backcountry.

Appalachian Trail Nutrition Survey

Thank you for participating in the Appalachian Trail Nutrition Survey. This is not a marketing study and we are not trying to sell you anything. I am a physician practicing near the Trail and a backpacker myself. At a recent Wilderness Medical Society meeting, several experts made recommendation on backpackers' nutritional needs. Someone asked if anyone knew what a long distance backpacker really ate. No one knew of any studies. This is an attempt to fill that void. With your help we hope to document the diet and nutrition practices of a large number of long distance hikers. We hope to publish the results. Your help completing this survey is <u>much</u> appreciated. Please <u>fill in the spaces or circle your answers</u>.

1) Would you describe your current hike as:
   A) Through hike
   B) Section of hike 7 days or more
   C) Section of hike less than 7 days

2) How many days have you been on the trail? ________ days

3) How many miles did you hike yesterday? ________ miles

4) Are you Male or Female ?

5) Hometown ____________________

6) Age ________ Weight ________ Height ________

7) Which best describes the major portion of your food supply:
   A) Purchased off the shelf at supermarket
   B) Freeze-dried purchased at outdoor specialty store
   C) Home dehydrated
   D) Military surplus (MREs)

8) How do you re-supply your food on this hike?
   A) Mail drops at towns along the trail
   B) Purchase at stores near the trail
   C) Carry everything (no need to re-supply)

9) How often do you eat at restaurants during this hike?
   A) Never
   B) Almost never (once a month)

C) Several times a month
D) Every chance I get (more than once a week)

10) Do you regularly take vitamins, nutritional supplements or herbal preparations? YES NO
If yes please specify

____

11) Do you occasionally eat wild foods (berries, plants, bugs, fish) along the trail? YES NO

12) In the past <u>week</u> how many servings of fruits or vegetables have you eaten?
________ svgs/wk

13) Have you ever "run out of food" or gone on short rations during this hike?
YES NO

14) On average, how much water do you consume each day? ________ quarts or liters/day

15) Please write down <u>everything</u> you have eaten in the past <u>24 hours</u>. Please include meals (breakfast, lunch, dinner) snacks and beverages. Record the amount and brand if possible. For example: 1 cup oatmeal with 2 teaspoons sugar and 1 tablespoon raisins, Kraft macaroni and cheese (whole box), Lipton noodle dinner (whole bag), 1 apple, handful of wild blueberries, Milky Way Bar (large), Gatorade mix (one quart). This is called a "24-hour diet recall" and is a standard tool among diet researchers. Please be as accurate and detailed as possible.

24 Hour Diet Recall:

Please include any comments or stories you may have regarding trail food. These may include such things as "best foods," "worst foods," unusual foods, recipes, or "food fantasies."

POPULAR AT TRAIL FOODS

This survey of AT hikers reveals many beliefs about food and nutrition observed in both the NOLS community and the backcountry nutrition classes I have taught in Wyoming. Overall, many hikers believe it is difficult to "eat healthy" while on the trail due to excessively processed foods and not enough fresh foods. While it is true that the processed grains and packaged meals that are most convenient in the backcountry are not the best nutritional choice for everyday living, there are many nutritious foods that can be taken into the backcountry to provide a balance of important nutrients. There are certainly nutritional tradeoffs that are discussed in several chapters of this book, and part of eating well in the backcountry includes understanding how to fuel your body well, given the limitations in a backcountry environment.

There were many comments in these surveys that reflect common misperceptions about the role of carbohydrates, fat, and protein in the backcountry. It is also interesting that many AT hikers take supplements while on the trail, but eat little or no fruits and vegetables and a lot of foods with calories but few nutrients, such as Pop-Tarts and candy bars. Many of the vegetarian hikers (especially vegans) found it difficult to resupply along the trail at grocery stores, especially in the smaller towns. (This may have changed since the survey was conducted.)

The goal of this book is to shed some light on the ways that nutrition can enhance a long backcountry adventure, such as hiking the Appalachian Trail. The first section of this book addresses each of the macronutrients in detail, and the list of nutrition myths and facts in chapter 13 is a good place to review many of these common misperceptions. The nutritional overview in appendix H is also helpful for a quick reference about the major nutrients.

The reported popular foods for trail snacks, meals, and beverages appear to be similar, based on NOLS rations and reports from other backcountry travelers. There are most certainly some regional differences in grocery store foods, and hikers who chose to resupply using mail drops seemed to have significantly different backcountry diets than those who chose to shop at grocery stores along the way. The following lists were compiled from the surveys to give an idea of what AT hikers eat and to share some of their food fantasies and thoughts about food.

TOP 10 SNACKS

Candy bars, especially Snickers
Cheese and cracker, packaged, some with peanut butter
Chex, cereal mix
Dried fruit and fruit leather
Granola bars
Jerky or Slim Jims
Little Debbie's cookies
Pop-Tarts
Sausage or pepperoni
Trail mix

TOP 10 OTHER FOODS

Bagels
Cheese
Lipton dinners
Macaroni and cheese
Oatmeal, instant
Pasta
Peanut butter
Ramen noodles
Soups

POPULAR TRAIL BEVERAGES (OTHER THAN WATER)

Coffee
Crystal Light
Gatorade
Hot chocolate
Powdered milk
Tang drink mixes
Tea

MOST COMMONLY CRAVED FOODS

Pizza—the number one fantasy
Chocolate
Cola
Fresh vegetables and fruit
Ice cream
Steak

MOST INTERESTING FOODS

- Assorted flavors of nutritional bars combined in a bag and melted together (in the sun) to form "an incredibly interesting and varied bar to pick at all week"
- Jelly tea: boiled water with jelly stirred in to taste
- Fruit leather and protein powder "so I can stick to my 40-30-30 plan on the trail—I cheat on all kinds of foods in town though (ice cream, bread)"
- Tabasco sauce added to peanut butter sandwich
- Peanut butter and canned frosting
- Snickers bar dipped in mayo
- Rattlesnake
- Frog legs
- Uncooked pancake batter (no stove—listed as a "worst food")

FOOD FANTASIES AND THOUGHTS

"Not long ago I ate a whole chicken, a calzone and a 12-cut pizza and although I could not physically eat more I was still hungry. At every road crossing I have to force myself not to run for food. I dream about food. For fun I go to supermarkets and look at food. My last through hike in '98 I lost 40 pounds."

"The old Thanksgiving dinner would be bliss."

"I went through US Army Ranger School so my perceptions of 'going hungry' or best/worst foods are warped. If it isn't an MRE I'm happy!"

"The whole time we were up north I craved and talked about good ol' mushy southern-style vegetables! Nothing beats green beans cooked in fat back!!"

"I ate Jack cheese—Kraft 'cause it never rots, which in a way should be a deterrent."

"Clif Bars, Power Bars all taste alike. I quit eating them when I noticed they look the same coming out as going in."

"Energy bars over the course of several days made a difference in my physical and mental well-being (tried various brands—Met Rx, Power Bar, Clif, Geni Soy)."

"I ate very little meat before the trip. Now I am a ravenous carnivore! I eat burgers and steaks in every town."

"I fantasize about dehydrated beer tablets."

"Reduced fat food is, well, dumb."

"I'm thinking more about food than ever. My appetite wasn't much at the beginning of the AT but now (105 days into it) I can't wait to eat . . . especially in town."

"I can never get enough food—I can't carry enough."

APPENDIX H

OVERVIEW OF BACKCOUNTRY NUTRITION BASICS

WHY TEACH NUTRITION IN THE FIELD?

Health and strength
Performance—energy and moods
Immune system
Good "EB"

IMPORTANT NUTRITION INFORMATION TO START THE TRIP

- Initially you will need to eat and drink more often to stay fueled and hydrated.
- As you build more muscle, you will store more glycogen (carbohydrate) and water and can go longer between fueling.
- Protein and iron needs may be higher while building muscle.
- You need to drink before you are thirsty and continue during and after exercise.
- At altitude, in hot climates, or during days of heavy exertion, appetite and thirst may be suppressed; you may need to force yourself to eat and drink.
- Be familiar with which foods in your ration are high in carbohydrate, protein, fat, and other important nutrients.
- Have an idea how many calories you need, and how much food you need to eat to get those calories.

OVERVIEW OF NUTRIENTS

ENERGY

- Calories measure the amount of energy we get from food.
- Energy keeps us warm and fuels us.
- Calorie needs are based on the energy we need for basic functions (e.g., breathing, thinking, and heartbeat), the digestion of nutrients, and physical activity.
- (There are tables in the energy chapter and appendix D to help you estimate basic energy needs.)

WATER

- Water is the most important nutrient in the backcountry.
- Do not assume water in the backcountry is safe to drink. Always use some method of disinfection (boiling, filters, tablets, etc.).
- Water provides no food energy, but it is essential for all body functions.
- Not getting enough water in the field can make you feel tired, lethargic, and crabby; affect how well your muscles work; and cause headaches and gastrointestinal problems (cramps, constipation, and bloating).
- When exercising in the backcountry, drink early and drink often.
- The exact amount of water you need to consume will vary depending on the activity and environment, but it should be at least 2 to 4 quarts daily. Two quarts may be enough for a mellow rest day, and 4 or 5 quarts on a more typically active day in the field.

RISK FACTORS FOR DEHYDRATION

Extreme heat, cold, and humidity
High altitude
High protein diet
High sodium diet
Vomiting and diarrhea
Infection and fever
Inadequate fluid intake

Medications
Laxatives
Diuretics, may include caffeine—varies according to use

SYMPTOMS OF DEHYDRATION

Weakness
Headache
Fatigue
Lethargy
Constipation
Mental confusion
Increased heart rate
Decreased urine output

Food also contributes to hydration status. If you eat less food for any reason (decreased appetite or illness), you need to drink more.

Make sure you are urinating regularly and the color is straw. Cold or high altitude may increase urination even if you are dehydrated. Some vitamins give urine a bright yellow color, so color is a less accurate measure of how well-hydrated you are. Basically, you don't want a trickle of dark urine or hours without producing any. Constipation, bloating, and stomach or muscle cramps are other signs that you may not be getting enough fluid.

CARBOHYDRATES

- Carbohydrates are the main energy source for exercise.
- Carbohydrates are the primary fuel for high intensity exercise and in hot, cold, and high-altitude environments.
- Carbohydrates are stored as glycogen in the liver (to fuel your brain and other cells) and in muscles (to fuel activity).
- Depleting muscle glycogen stores leads to muscle weakness, fatigue, and ultimately the inability to continue exercise (aka "hitting the wall").
- Depleting liver glycogen causes low blood sugar symptoms (aka "bonking").

SYMPTOMS OF HYPOGLYCEMIA (LOW BLOOD SUGAR)

Dizziness
Confusion
Disorientation
Irritability
Weakness
Fatigue
Headaches
Extreme hunger
Anxiety
Fast heartbeat
Sweating
Shaking
Impaired vision

- Well-trained muscle can store 20 to 50 percent more glycogen than untrained muscle.
- Exercise lasting longer than ninety minutes benefits from carbohydrate intake (food or drinks) to keep muscles and brain fueled.
- There is no substitute for high carbohydrate meals at dinner and breakfast.
- Replenishing glycogen stores before and after exercise is crucial, in addition to carbohydrate intake during exercise.
- Dietary fiber is important to keep bowel movements regular, control blood sugar levels, and to increase feeling of fullness. In the long term, fiber may lower the risk of several chronic diseases.
- Eating more carbohydrate and less fat means eating more food to get enough calories for exercise. (This is good knowledge for weight-conscious students who do not normally eat a vegetarian-type diet.)
- The "magic window" for replacing carbs after a day in the field is 15 to 30 minutes after exercise. Ideally postexercise food includes carbohydrate plus some protein.
- Eating high fat meals during or after exercise can lead to inadequate carbohydrate intake (you fill up before getting enough carbs).

- The recommendations for carbohydrates during exercise lasting more than ninety minutes is 30 to 60 grams per hour ($\frac{1}{4}$ cup of chocolate covered raisins 5 33 grams of carbohydrates. (See appendix C for other choices). A snack at water breaks is probably the best way to do this in the field. Keeping an extra water bottle with drink mix is also helpful.
- High carbohydrate diets can reduce cortisol levels. Cortisol is a hormone that may suppress immune function and contribute to overtraining syndrome common among endurance athletes.

PROTEIN

- Proteins are made up of amino acids. Our bodies can make all but nine of the twenty amino acids. The nine we cannot make are called essential and must come from our diet.
- Protein (amino acids) has many functions: grow and repair body tissues; provide structure for muscle, bone, tendons, ligaments, and organs; form enzymes, hormones, and antibodies (immune system); maintain fluid and electrolyte balance and acid-base balance; transport fats, minerals, and oxygen; play a role in blood clotting; and provide some energy.
- Protein Recommendations:

  Grams of Protein per Pound of Body Weight

Current RDA, sedentary adult	= .4
Recreational exerciser, adult	= .5 to .75
Competitive athlete, adult	= .6 to .9*
Adult building muscle mass	= .7 to .9
Growing teenage athlete	= .8 to .9

  *No evidence that more than .9 provides any benefits.
- Enough protein is essential for health and athletic performance. Excess protein is stored as fat (just like excess carbohydrates and fat).
- Adequate protein (combined with exercise) is required to build muscle mass. Excessive protein intake does not increase muscle mass.

- Complete proteins, found in animal foods (meat, chicken, fish, eggs, and dairy) and soybeans, contain all of the essential amino acids in the proper amounts to form new proteins.
- Plant proteins other than soy (nuts, seeds, grains, beans, and legumes) may be combined throughout the day to provide the necessary amino acids. They do not need to be combined at each meal or snack.

FAT

- Fat is a major energy source, especially for low intensity and prolonged physical activity.
- Burning fat efficiently requires some carbohydrate and plenty of oxygen.
- If exercise is intense or occurs in an extreme environment (hot, cold, or high altitude), fat is not the main fuel (burning carbohydrates is more efficient and requires less oxygen).
- Avoiding fat in the field can make it difficult to get enough calories to meet energy needs (fat yields 9 calories per gram, versus 4 calories per gram for protein and carbohydrate).
- Trained athletes can use fat at a higher intensity level than untrained athletes.
- Adjusting to more fat, fiber, or natural fruit sugar (fructose) may initially cause gastrointestinal distress (abdominal cramps, diarrhea, and nausea).
- The amount of fat consumed in the field may be higher than recommendations for the general public due to high levels of physical activity and higher calorie needs. This is acceptable, especially for the more beneficial fats common in many backcountry foods.

General Recommendations for Fat Intake

Lower limit for intake = 15 percent of total calories
Upper limit for intake = 30 percent of total calories
Saturated fat = 0 to 10 percent of total calories

VITAMINS AND MINERALS

- Vitamins and minerals provide no energy (calories) but are essential for all bodily functions.
- Eating enough calories to meet backcountry needs, including a variety of foods, should be enough to prevent any major nutrient deficiencies.
- Review the tables in chapter 6 for information about the functions, amounts needed, and food sources of various vitamins and minerals.
- Antioxidants may be important in the backcountry to mitigate the effects of oxidative stress. In addition to the vitamins A, C, and E and the mineral selenium, there are thousands of plant compounds (phytonutrients) that exert antioxidant effects. Eat a variety of nuts, seeds, grains, beans, legumes, and dried fruits and vegetables to provide protective macro- and micronutrients and phytonutrients.
- Deficiency symptoms listed in the vitamin and mineral tables have multiple causes. Not getting enough carbohydrate (or timing intake poorly, so low blood sugar results), protein, or water can cause many of these effects.
- For prolonged trips in extreme environments, a multivitamin and mineral supplement may be good "insurance" for adequate intakes.

REFERENCES

Introduction

Pearson, C. *NOLS Cookery*, 5th ed. Mechanicsburg, PA: Stackpole Books, 2004.

Chapter 1—Energy

Ainslie, P. N., I.T. Campbell, K. N. Frayn, S. M. Humphreys, D. P. MacLaren, T. Reilly, and K. R. Westerterp. August 2002. Energy balance, metabolism, hydration, and performance during strenuous hill walking: The effect of age. *Journal of Applied Physiology*. 93(2):714–23.

Backpacking Light Magazine. www.backpackinglight.com.

Benardot, D. 2007. *Advanced Sports Nutrition*. Champaign, IL: Human Kinetics.

Girard Eberle, S. 2007. *Endurance Sports Nutrition*, 2nd ed. Champaign, IL: Human Kinetics.

Go Lite. www.golite.com.

Howley, M. 2002. *NOLS Nutrition Field Guide*. Lander, WY: National Outdoor Leadership School.

McArdle, W., F. Katch, and V. Katch. 2005. *Sports & Exercise Nutrition*, 2nd ed. Baltimore, MD: Lippincott Williams & Wilkins.

Sample day calculations. Based on activity calculator at www.caloriesperhour.com.

Sample menu analysis. ESHA Food Processor for Windows version 7.9., ESHA Research: Salem, OR, 2002.

Williams, M. 1999. *Nutrition for Health, Fitness and Sport*, 5th ed. Boston, MA: WCB McGraw-Hill.

Chapter 2—Water

Benardot, D. 2006. *Advanced Sports Nutrition*. Champaign, IL: Human Kinetics.

Casa, D. J., L. E. Armstrong, S. K. Hillman, S. J. Montain, R. V. Reiff, B. S. Rich, W. O. Roberts, and J. A. Stone. April 2000. National Athletic Trainers' Association position statement: Fluid replacement for athletes. *Journal of Athletic Training*. 35(2):212–224.

Cheuvront, S. N., R. Carter, J. W. Castellani, and M. N. Sawka. November 2005. Hypohydration impairs endurance exercise performance in temperate but not cold air. *Journal of Applied Physiology*. 99(5):1972–6.

Clark, N. 1997. *Nancy Clark's Sports Nutrition Guidebook*, 2nd ed. Champaign, IL: Human Kinetics.

Colgan, M. 1993. *Optimum Sports Nutrition: Your Competitive Edge*. NY: Advanced Research Press.

Coyle, E., D. Costill, and W. Fink. 1978. Gastric emptying rates for selected athletic drinks. *Research Quarterly* (49):119–124.

Girard Eberle, S. 2007. *Endurance Sports Nutrition*, 2nd ed. Champaign, IL: Human Kinetics.

Godek, S. F., A. R. Bartolozzi, and J. J. Godek. April 2005. Sweat rate and fluid turnover in American football players compared with runners in a hot and humid environment. *British Journal of Sports Medicine*. 39(4):205–11.

Howley, M. 2002. *NOLS Nutrition Field Guide*. Lander, WY: National Outdoor Leadership School.

Jung, A. P., P. A. Bishop, A. Al-Nawwas, and R. B. Dale. June 2005. Influence of hydration and electrolyte supplementation on incidence and time to onset of exercise-associated muscle cramps. *Journal of Athletic Training*. 40(2):71–75.

Kenny, G. P., A. A. Chen, C. E. Johnston, J. S. Thoden, and G. G. Giesbrecht. 1997. Intense exercise increases the post-exercise threshold for sweating. *European Journal of Applied Physiology and Occupational Physiology*. 76(2):116–21.

Maresh, C. M., C. L. Gabaree-Boulant, L. E. Armstrong, D. A. Judelson, J. R. Hoffman, J. W. Castellani, R. W. Kenefick, M. F. Bergeron, and D. J. Casa. July 2004. Effect of hydration status on thirst, drinking, and related hormonal responses during low-intensity exercise in the heat. *Journal of Applied Physiology*. 97(1):39–44.

Martin, W. F., L. H. Cerundolo, M. A. Pikosky, P. C. Gaine, C. M. Maresh, L. E. Armstrong, D. R. Bolster, and N. R. Rodriguez. April 2006. Effects of dietary protein intake on indexes of hydration. *Journal of the American Dietetic Association*. 106(4):587–9.

Montain, S. J., S. N. Cheuvront, and M. N. Sawka. February 2006. Exercise associated hyponatremia: Quantitative analysis to understand the aetiology. *British Journal of Sports Medicine.* 40(2):98-105; discussion 98–105.

Morris, J. G., M. E. Nevill, D. Thompson J. Collie, and C. Williams. May 2003. The influence of a 6.5% carbohydrate-electrolyte solution on performance of prolonged intermittent high-intensity running at 30 degrees C. *Journal of Sports Science and Medicine.* 21(5):371–81.

Mündel, T., J. King, E. Collacott, and D. A. Jones. 2006. Drink temperature influences fluid intake and endurance capacity in men during exercise in a hot, dry environment. *Experimental Physiology.* 91(5):925–33.

Murray, B. Sports drinks: Myths and facts. Gatorade Sports Science Institute. www.gssiweb.com/Article_Detail.aspx?articleid=573&level=2&topic=1

Sawka, M. N., S. N. Cheuvront, and R. Carter. June 2005. Human water needs. *Nutrition Review* 63(6 Pt 2):S30–9.

Schimelpfenig, T. (Curriculum Director, WMI of NOLS). Updated July 2006. Hydration: WMI curriculum enrichment. www.nols.edu/wmi/curriculum_updates/archive/041103_hydration.shtml

Shirreffs, S. M. June 2005. The importance of good hydration for work and exercise performance. *Nutrition Reviews.* 63(6 Pt 2): S14–21.

Sizer, F., and E. Whitney. 1997. *Nutrition Concepts and Controversies,* 7th ed. Belmont, CA: West/Wadsworth International Thomson Publishing Company.

Thermal and Mountain Medicine Division, U.S. Army Research Institute of Environmental Medicine, Natick, MA 01760-5007, USA. michael.sawka@us.army.mil

Tilton, B. As the stomach churns: A backpacker's guide to the runs. www.nols.edu/wmi/articles/archive/stomach.shtml.

Vallier, J. M., F. Grego, F. Basset, R. Lepers, T. Bernard, and J. Brisswalter. April 2005. Effect of fluid ingestion on neuromuscular function during prolonged cycling exercise. *British Journal of Sports Medicine.* 39(4):e17. E.A. 3162.

Water disinfection information: www.epa.gov/safewater/faq/emerg.html.

Wilerson, J. 2001. *Medicine for Mountaineering and other Wilderness Activities,* 5th ed. Seattle, WA: The Mountaineers Books.

Williams, M. 1999. *Nutrition for Health, Fitness and Sport,* 5th ed. Boston, MA: WCB McGraw-Hill.

Wingo, J. E., D. J. Casa, E. M. Berger, W. O. Dellis, J. C. Knight, and J. M. McClung. June 2004. Influence of a pre-exercise glycerol hydration beverage on performance and physiologic function during mountain-bike races in the heat. *Journal of Athletic Training.* 39(2):169–175.

Chapter 3—Carbohydrates

Benardot, D. 2006. *Advanced Sports Nutrition*. Champaign, IL: Human Kinetics.

Benson, J., and W. Askew. 1999. Nutrition for athletes. *Lifestyles Medicine.* MA: Blackwell Science, 182–185.

Brun, M., C. Dumortier, J. Fedou, and J. F. Mercier. 2001. Exercise hypoglycemia in nondiabetic subjects. Masson, Paris. 27(2):92.

Burke, L. M., A. B. Loucks, and N. Broad. July 2006. Energy and carbohydrate for training and recovery. *Journal of Sports Science.* 24(7):675–85.

Burke, L. M., G. R. Collier, E. M. Broad, P. G. Davis, D. T. Martin, A. J. Sanigorski, and M. Hargreaves. September 2003. Effect of alcohol intake on muscle glycogen storage after prolonged exercise. *Journal of Applied Physiology.* 95(3):983–90.

Clark, N. 1997. *Nancy Clark's Sports Nutrition Guidebook*, 2nd ed. Champaign, IL: Human Kinetics.

Colgan, M. 1993. *Optimum Sports Nutrition: Your Competitive Edge*. NY: Advanced Research Press.

Davis, J. M., and A. Brown. SSE #80: Carbohydrates, Hormones, and endurance performance. *Sports Science Exchange.* 14(1).

Girard Eberle, S. 2007. *Endurance Sports Nutrition*, 2nd ed. Champaign, IL: Human Kinetics.

Howley, M. 2002. *NOLS Nutrition Field Guide*. Lander, WY: National Outdoor Leadership School.

Hu, Y, G. Block, E. P. Norkus, J. D. Morrow, M. Dietrich, and M. Hudes. July 2006. Relations of glycemic index and glycemic load with plasma oxidative stress markers. *American Journal of Clinical Nutrition.* 84(1):70–6; quiz 266–7.

Jackson, D., J. Davis, and M. Broadwell. 1995. Effects of carbohydrate feeding on fatigue during intermittent high-intensity exercise in males and females. *Medicine and Science in Sports and Exercise.* 27(suppl):S223.

Passias, T. C., G. S. Meneilly, and I. B. Mekjavi. March 1996. Effect of hypoglycemia on thermoregulatory responses. *Journal of Applied Physiology*. 80(3):1021–32.

Siu, P., and S. Wong. 2004. Use of the glycemic index: Effects on feeding patterns and exercise performance. *Journal of Physiological Anthropology and Applied Human Science.* 23(1):1–6.

Sizer, F., and E. Whitney. 1997. *Nutrition Concepts and Controversies*, 7th ed. Belmont, CA: West/Wadsworth International Thomson Publishing Company.

Walberg Rankin, J. 1994. SSE #64: Glycemic index and exercise metabolism. *Sports Science Exchange.* 80(1).

Williams, M. 1999. *Nutrition for Health, Fitness and Sport*, 5th ed. Boston, MA: WCB McGraw-Hill.

Chapter 4—Protein

Antinoro, L. Oct. 2003. Protein packs powerful punch: Are you getting enough for optimal health? *Environmental Nutrition Newsletter*. 26(10).

Benardot, D. 2006. *Advanced Sports Nutrition*. Champaign, IL: Human Kinetics.

Clark, N. 1997. *Nancy Clark's Sports Nutrition Guidebook*, 2nd ed. Champaign, IL: Human Kinetics.

Flakoll, P. J., T. Judy, K. Flinn, C. Carr, and S. Flinn. March 2004. Postexercise protein supplementation improves health and muscle soreness during basic military training in Marine recruits. *Journal of Applied Physiology*. 96(3):951–6.

Girard Eberle, S. 2007. *Endurance Sports Nutrition*, 2nd ed. Champaign, IL: Human Kinetics.

Howley, M. 2002. *NOLS Nutrition Field Guide*. Lander, WY: National Outdoor Leadership School.

Lemon, P. W. 2000. Beyond the zone: Protein needs of active individuals. *Journal of the American College of Nutrition* 19(5 Suppl): 513S–521S.

Martin, W. F., L. H. Cerundolo, M. A. Pikosky, P. C. Gaine, C. M. Maresh, L. E. Armstrong, D. R. Bolster, and N. R. Rodriguez. April 2006. Effects of dietary protein intake on indexes of hydration. *Journal of the American Dietetic Association*. 106(4):587–9.

Nutritional Needs in Cold and in High-altitude Environments. 1996. Washington, D.C.: National Academy Press, 39.

Sizer, F., and E. Whitney. 1997. *Nutrition Concepts and Controversies*, 7th ed. Belmont, CA: West/Wadsworth International Thomson Publishing Company.

Williams, M. 1999. *Nutrition for Health, Fitness and Sport*, 5th ed. Boston, MA: WCB McGraw-Hill.

Zachwieja, J. 2004. Gatorade Sports Science Institute statement on new sports drink research regarding protein during exercise. *Gatorade Sports Science Institute*. www.gssiweb.com/Article_Detail.aspx?articleid=665&level=2&topic=1

Chapter 5—Fat

Girard Eberle, S. 2007. *Endurance Sports Nutrition*, 2nd ed. Champaign, IL: Human Kinetics.

Howley, M. 2002. *NOLS Nutrition Field Guide*. Lander, WY: National Outdoor Leadership School.

König, D., A. Berg, C. Weinstock, J. Keul, and H. Northoff. 1997. Essential fatty acids, immune function, and exercise. *Exercise Immunology Review*. 3:1–31.

Sizer, F., and E. Whitney. 1997. *Nutrition Concepts and Controversies*, 7th ed. Belmont, CA: West/Wadsworth International Thomson Publishing Company.

Smith, S., L. de Jonge, J. Zachwieja, H. Roy, T. Nguyen, J. Rood, M. Windhauser, and G. Bray. 2000. Fat and carbohydrate balances during adaptation to a high-fat diet. *American Journal of Clinical Nutrition* 71:450–7.

Venkatraman, J. T., J. Leddy, and D. Pendergast. July 2000. Dietary fats and immune status in athletes: Clinical implications. *Medicine and Science in Sports and Exercise.* 32(7 Suppl):S389–95.

Williams, M. 1999. *Nutrition for Health, Fitness and Sport*, 5th ed. Boston, MA: WCB McGraw-Hill.

Chapter 6—Vitamins, Minerals and Phytonutrients

Antinoro, L. 2005. A radical notion: Maybe antioxidants can't protect us after all. *Environmental Nutrition Newsletter*. 28(3).

Benardot, D. 2006. *Advanced Sports Nutrition*. Champaign, IL: Human Kinetics.

Blumberg, J., P. Clarkson, A. Goldfarb, R. Jenkins, and L. L. Ji. 1994. SSE Roundtable #15: Exercise, nutrition and free radicals: What's the connection? *Sports Science Exchange*. 5(1).

Chu, Y. F., J. Sun, X. Wu, and R. H. Liu. November 2002. Antioxidant and antiproliferative activities of common vegetables. *Journal of Agricultural and Food Chemistry.* 50(23):6910–6.

Dietz, J., and J. Erdman. 1989. Effects of thermal processing upon vitamins and proteins in foods. *Nutrition Today*. 24(4):6–5.

Driskell, J., and I. Wolinsky. 1999. *Macroelements, Water, and Electrolytes in Sports Nutrition*. New York: CRC Press.

Girard Eberle, S. 2007. *Endurance Sports Nutrition*, 2nd ed. Champaign, IL: Human Kinetics.

Gropper, S., J. Smith, and J. Groff. 2005. *Advanced Nutrition and Human Metabolism*, 4th ed. Belmont, CA: Thomson Wadsworth.

Howley, M. 2002. *NOLS Nutrition Field Guide*. Lander, WY: National Outdoor Leadership School.

Lips, P. September 2006. Vitamin D physiology. *Prog Biophys Mol Biol.* 92(1):4–8.

Nutritional Needs in Cold and in High-Altitude Environments. Washington, D.C.: National Academy Press, 39.

Powers, S., L. Ji, and C. Leeuwenburgh. 1999. Exercise training-induced alterations in skeletal muscle antioxidant capacity: A brief review. *Medicine and Science in Sports and Exercise.* 31(7):987–97.

Powers, S., L. Ji, and C. Leeuwenburgh. May 2000. Expert panel shuns antioxidant supplements, pushes food sources. *Environmental Nutrition Newsletter of Food, Nutrition and Health.* 23(5).

Rall, L., and S. Meydani. 1999. Vitamin E, vitamin C, and immune response: Recent advances. *Nutrition and Immune Function.* Washington, D.C.: National Academy Press, 289–303.

Sizer, F., and E. Whitney. 1997. *Nutrition Concepts and Controversies*, 7th ed. Belmont, CA: West/Wadsworth International Thomson Publishing Company.

Tiidus, P., and M. Houston. 1995. Vitamin E status and response to exercise training. *American College of Sports Medicine*. 20(1):12–23.

Vinson, J., L. Zubik, P. Bose, N. Samman, and J. Proch. Dried fruits: Excellent in vitro and in vivo antioxidants. *Journal of the American College of Nutrition*. www.jacn.org/cgi/content/abstract/24/1/44.

Williams, M. 1999. *Nutrition for Health, Fitness and Sport*, 5th ed. Boston, MA: WCB McGraw-Hill.

Wright, H. June 2007. Vitamin D may help you dodge cancer: How to be sure you get enough. *Environmental Nutrition Newsletter*. 30(6).

Chapter 7—Food and Mood

Adam, T. C., and E. S. Epel. July 2007. Stress, eating and the reward system. *Physiology and Behavior*. 91(4):449–58.

Garner, D.M. 1997. Psychoeducational principles in the treatment of eating disorders. *Handbook for Treatment of Eating Disorders*. D.M. Garner and P.E. Garfinkel, eds. New York: Guilford Press, 145–177.

Black, P.H. 2006. The inflammatory consequences of psychologic stress: Relationship to insulin resistance, obesity, atherosclerosis and diabetes mellitus, type II. *Medical Hypotheses*. 67(4):879-91. Epub June 15, 2006.

Geiselman, P. J. December 1996. Control of food intake: A physiologically complex, motivated behavioral system. *Endocrinology and Metabolism Clinics of North America*. 25(4):815–29.

Gibson, E. L. August 2006. Emotional influences on food choice: Sensory, physiological and psychological pathways. *Physiology and Behavior*. 89(1):53–61.

Hill, A. J. May 2007. The psychology of food craving. *Proceedings of the Nutrition Society*. 66(2):277–85.

Levitsky, D. A. April 2002. Putting behavior back into feeding behavior: A tribute to George Collier. *Appetite*. 38(2):143–8.

Lowe, M. R., and A. S. Levine. May 2005. Eating motives and the controversy over dieting: Eating less than needed versus less than wanted. *Obesity Research*. 13(5): 797–806.

Lowe, M. R., and M. L. Butryn. July 2007. Hedonic hunger: A new dimension of appetite? *Physiology and Behavior*. 91(4):432–9.

Oliver, G., J. Wardle, and E. L. Gibson. November–December 2000. Stress and food choice: A laboratory study. *Psychosomatic Medicine*. 62(6): 853–65.

Pecoraro, N., F. Reyes, F. Gomez, A. Bhargava, and M. F. Dallman. August 2004. Chronic stress promotes palatable feeding, which reduces signs of stress: Feedforward and feedback effects of chronic stress. *Endocrinology*. 145(8):3754–62.

Phillips, W. J. July 1994. Starvation and survival: Some military considerations. *Military Medicine.* 159(7):513–6.

Plata-Salamán, C. R. 1991. Regulation of hunger and satiety in man. *Journal of Digestive Diseases.* 9(5):253–68.

Polivy, J. June 1996. Psychological consequences of food restriction. *Journal of the American Dietetic Association.* 96(6):589-92; quiz 593–4.

Quinlan, P., J. Lane, and L. Aspinall. November 1997. Effects of hot tea, coffee and water ingestion on physiological responses and mood: The role of caffeine, water and beverage type. *Psychopharmacology (Berl).* 134(2):164–73.

Scott, D., J. A. Rycroft, J. Aspen, C. Chapman, and B. Brown. April 2004. The effect of drinking tea at high altitude on hydration status and mood. *European Journal of Applied Physiology.* 91(4):493–8.

Somer, E. 1999. *Food and Mood,* 2nd ed. New York, NY: Henry Holt and Co.

Ulrich-Lai, Y. M., M. M. Ostrander, I. M. Thomas, B. A. Packard, A. R. Furay, C. M. Dolgas, D. C. Van Hooren, H. F. Figueiredo, N. K. Mueller, D. C. Choi, and J. P. Herman. April 2007. Daily limited access to sweetened drink attenuates hypothalamic-pituitary-adrenocortical axis stress responses. *Endocrinology.* 148(4):1823–34. Epub January 4, 2007.

Yun, A. J., and J. D. Doux. 2007. Unhappy meal: How our need to detect stress may have shaped our preferences for taste. *Medical Hypotheses.* Epub ahead of print March 19.

Chapter 8—Health and Illness

Acheson, D. W., and S. Luccioli. April 2004. Microbial-gut interactions in health and disease. *Best Practice and Research Clinical Gastroenterology.* 18(2):387–404.

Anderson, S., and C. J. H. Johnson. 2000. Expedition health and safety: A risk assessment. *Journal of the Royal Society of Medicine.* 93:557–562.

Boulware, D. R., W. W. Forgey, and W. J. Martin. March 2003. Medical risks of wilderness hiking. *American Journal of Medicine.* 114(4):288–93.

Glazer, J. L. June 2005. Management of heatstroke and heat exhaustion. *American Family Physician.* 71(11):2133–40.

König, D., A. Berg, C. Weinstock, J. Keul, and H. Northoff. 1997. Essential fatty acids, immune function, and exercise. *Exercise Immunology Review.* 3:1–31.

Neville, K. August 2007. Probiotics promise better health: Put a few billion of them on your plate. *Environmental Nutrition Newsletter.* 30(8).

Nieman, D. C. October 2000. Special feature for the Olympics: Effects of exercise on the immune system: Exercise effects on systemic immunity. *Immunology and Cell Biology.* 78(5):496–501.

Venkatraman, J. T., and D. R. Pendergast. 2002. Effect of dietary intake on immune function in athletes. *American College of Sports Medicine.* 32(5):323–37.

Venkatraman, J. T., J. Leddy, and D. Pendergast. July 2000. Dietary fats and immune status in athletes: Clinical implications. *Medicine and Science in Sports and Exercise.* 32(7 Suppl):S389–95.

Zareie, M., K. Johnson-Henry, J. Jury, P. C. Yang, B. Y. Ngan, D. M. McKay, J. D. Soderholm, M. H. Perdue, and P. M. Sherman. November 2006. Probiotics prevent bacterial translocation and improve intestinal barrier function in rats following chronic psychological stress. *Gut.* 55(11):1553–60.

Chapter 9—Special Environments

Anand, I., and Y. Chandrashekhar. 1996. Fluid metabolism at high altitudes. *Nutritional Needs in Cold and in High-Altitude Environments.* Washington, D.C.: National Academy Press, 331–356.

Beard, J. 1996. Macronutrient deficiency states and thermoregulation in cold. *Nutritional Needs in Cold and in High-Altitude Environments.* Washington, D.C.: National Academy Press, 245–256.

Benardot, D. *Advanced Sports Nutrition.* Champaign, IL: Human Kinetics, 2006.

Burstein, R., A. W. Coward, W. E. Askew, K. Carmel, C. Irving, O. Shpilberg, D. Moran, A. Pikarsky, G. Ginot, M. Sawyer R. Golan, and Y. Epstein. December 1996. Energy expenditure variations in soldiers performing military activities under cold and hot climate conditions. *Military Medicine.* 161(12):750–4.

Casa, D. J. July 1999. Exercise in the heat I: Fundamentals of thermal physiology, performance implications, and dehydration. *Journal of Athletic Training.* 34(3):246–52.

Casa, D. J. July 1999. Exercise in the heat II: Critical concepts in rehydration, exertional heat illnesses, and maximizing athletic performance. *Journal of Athletic Training.* 34(3):253–62.

Castellani, J. W., A. J. Young, D. W. Degroot, D. A. Stulz, B. S. Cadarette, S. G. Rhind, J. Zamecnik, P. N. Shek, M. N. Sawka. March 2001. Thermoregulation during cold exposure after several days of exhaustive exercise. *Journal of Applied Physiology.* 90(3):939–46.

Chao, W. H., E. A. Askew, D. E. Roberts, S. M. Wood and J. B. Perkins JB. 1999. Oxidative stress in humans during work at moderate altitude. *Journal of Nutrition.* 129:2009–12.

Driskell, J., and I. Wolinsky. 1999. *Macroelements, Water, and Electrolytes in Sports Nutrition.* New York: CRC Press.

Dunagan, N., J. E. Greenleaf, and C. J. Cisar. December 1998. Thermoregulatory effects of caffeine ingestion during submaximal exercise in men. *Aviation, Space, and Environmental Medicine Journal.* 69(12):1178–81.

Freund, B., and M. Swaka. 1996. Influence of cold stress on human fluid balance. *Nutritional Needs in Cold and in High-Altitude Environments*. Washington, D.C.: National Academy Press, 161–79.

Girard Eberle, S. 2007. *Endurance Sports Nutrition*, 2nd ed. Champaign, IL: Human Kinetics.

Gonzalez, R. R., and L. A. Blanchard. August 1998. Thermoregulatory responses to cold transients: Effects of menstrual cycle in resting women. *Journal of Applied Physiology*. 85(2):543–53.

Howley, M. 2002. *NOLS Nutrition Field Guide*. Lander, WY: National Outdoor Leadership School.

Jequier, E. 1993. Body weight regulation in humans: The importance of nutrient balance. *News In Physiological Sciences*. 8:273–77.

Castellani, J. W., C. O'Brien, C. Baker-Fulco, M. N. Sawka, and A. J. Young. 2001. *Sustaining Health and Performance in Cold Weather Operations*. Natick, MA: U.S. Army Research Institute of Environmental Medicine.

Jones, P., and I. Lee. 1996. Macronutrient requirements for work in cold environments. *Nutritional Needs in Cold and in High-Altitude Environments*. Washington, D.C.: National Academy Press, 189–202.

Kenefick, R. W., N. V. Mahood, M. P. Hazzard, T. J. Quinn and J. W. Castellani. August 2004. Hypohydration effects on thermoregulation during moderate exercise in the cold. *European Journal of Applied Physiology*. 92(4-5):565–70.

Links Nerín, M. A., J. Palop, J. A. Montaño, J. R. Morandeira, and M. Vázquez. 2006. Acute mountain sickness: Influence of fluid intake. *Wilderness and Environmental Medicine Journal*. 17(4):215–20.

Maresh, C. M., C. L Gabaree-Boulant, L. E. Armstrong, D. A. Judelson, J. R. Hoffman, J. W. Castellani, R. W. Kenefick, M. F. Bergeron, and D. J. Casa. July 2004. Effect of hydration status on thirst, drinking, and related hormonal responses during low-intensity exercise in the heat. *Journal of Applied Physiology*. 97(1):39–44.

Reynolds, R. D., J. A. Lickteig, M. P. Howard, and P. A. Deuster. 1998. Intakes of high fat and high carbohydrate foods by humans increased with exposure to increasing altitude during an expedition to Mt. Everest. *Journal of Nutrition*. 128(1):50–55.

Reynolds, R. 1996. Effects of cold and altitude on vitamin and mineral requirements. *Nutritional Needs in Cold and in High-Altitude Environments*. Washington, D.C.: National Academy Press, 231–2.

Savourey, G., and J. Bittel. 1994. Cold thermoregulatory changes induced by sleep deprivation in men. *European Journal of Applied Physiology and Occupational Physiology*. 69(3):216–20.

Scott, D., J. A. Rycroft, J. Aspen, C. Chapman, and B. Brown. April 2004. The effect of drinking tea at high altitude on hydration status and mood. *European Journal of Applied Physiology.* 91(4):493–8.

Sridharan, K., S. Ranganathan, A. K. Mukherjee, M. L. Kumria, and P. Vats. 2004. Vitamin status of high altitude (3660 m) acclimatized human subjects during consumption of tinned rations. *Wilderness and Environmental Medicine Journal*. 15(2):95–101.

Usariem Technical Note 94-2. February 1994. *Medical Problems In High Mountain Environments: A Handbook For Medical Officers.* Natick, MA: U.S. Army Research Institute of Environmental Medicine.

Westerterp, K. R. 2001. Energy and water balance at high altitude. *News Physiology and Science.* 16.

Williams, M. 1999. *Nutrition for Health, Fitness and Sport*, 5th ed. Boston, MA: WCB McGraw-Hill.

Wingo, J. E., D. J. Casa, E. M. Berger, W. O. Dellis, J. C. Knight, and J. M. McClung. June 2004. Influence of a pre-exercise glycerol hydration beverage on performance and physiologic function during mountain-bike races in the heat. *Journal of Athletic Training.* 39(2):169–75.

Young, A., M. Sawka, and K. Pandolf. 1996. Physiology of cold exposure. *Nutritional Needs in Cold and in High-Altitude Environments.* Washington, D.C.: National Academy Press, 127–47.

Chapter 10—Teens

Bar-Or, O., S. Barr, M. Bergeron, R. Carey, P. Clarkson, L. Houtkooper, A. Rivera-Brown, T. Rowland, and S. Steen. 1997. SSE Roundtable #30: Youth in sport: Nutritional needs. *Sports Science Exchange.* 8(4).

Benardot, D. 2006. *Advanced Sports Nutrition.* Champaign, IL: Human Kinetics.

Inbar, O., N. Morris, Y. Epstein, and G. Gass. November 2004. Comparison of thermoregulatory responses to exercise in dry heat among prepubertal boys, young adults and older males. *Experimental Physiology.* 89(6):691–700.

Williams, M. 1999. *Nutrition for Health, Fitness and Sport*, 5th ed. Boston, MA: WCB McGraw-Hill.

Chapter 11—Special Diets

Girard Eberle, S. 2007. *Endurance Sports Nutrition*, 2nd ed. Champaign, IL: Human Kinetics.

Howley, M. 2002. *NOLS Nutrition Field Guide.* Lander, WY: National Outdoor Leadership School.

Kraehenbuhl, J. P., E. Pringault, M. R. Neutra. December 1997. Review article: Intestinal epithelia and barrier functions. *Alimentary Pharmacology and Therapeutics.* 11 Suppl 3:3–8; discussion 8–9.

Meerschaert, C. M. July 2007. Food allergy: A look at traditional and complementary diagnosis and treatment. *Today's Dietitian*. 9(7):40–43.

Nutritional yeast. en.wikipedia.org/wiki/Nutritional_yeast

Sicherer, S. H. 1998. Food allergy testing: Questions and answers. *Food Allergy News*. 7(4). The Food Allergy and Anaphylaxis Network. www.foodallergy.org

Sizer, F., and E. Whitney. 1997. *Nutrition Concepts and Controversies*, 7th ed. Belmont, CA: West/Wadsworth International Thomson Publishing Company.

Venderley, A. M., and W. W. Campbell. 2006. Vegetarian diets: Nutritional considerations for athletes. *American Journal of Sports Medicine*. 36(4):293–305.

Vickerstaff Jonega, J. M. July 2007. Food allergies: The immune response. *Today's Dietitian*. 9(7):12–16.

INDEX

Page numbers in italics indicate sidebars and tables.

C

P

Q

R

S

W

ABOUT THE AUTHOR

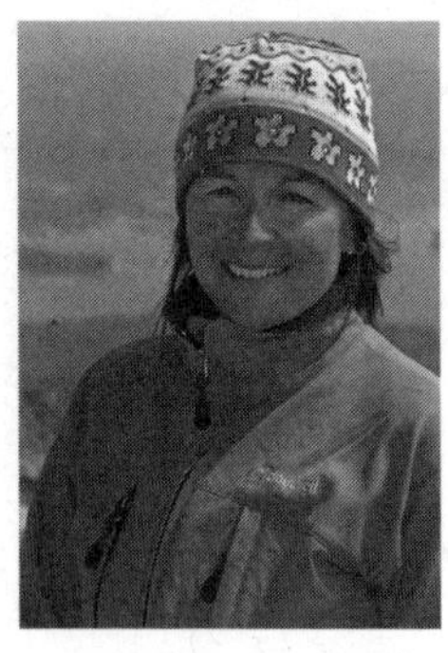

Mary Howley Ryan, MS, RD, is a dietitian, accomplished backcountry cook, and graduate of a NOLS Absaroka Backpacking course. She lives in Jackson, Wyoming, where she owns her own business, Beyond Broccoli Nutrition Counseling.